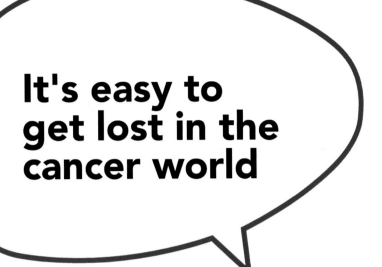

It's easy to get lost in the cancer world

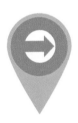

Let NCCN Guidelines for Patients® be your guide

✓ Step-by-step guides to the cancer care options likely to have the best results

✓ Based on treatment guidelines used by health care providers worldwide

✓ Designed to help you discuss cancer treatment with your doctors

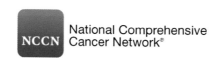

National Comprehensive
Cancer Network®

NCCN Guidelines for Patients® are developed by the National Comprehensive Cancer Network® (NCCN®)

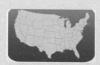

NCCN

✓ An alliance of leading cancer centers across the United States devoted to patient care, research, and education

Cancer centers that are part of NCCN:
NCCN.org/cancercenters

NCCN Clinical Practice Guidelines in Oncology (NCCN Guidelines®)

✓ Developed by doctors from NCCN cancer centers using the latest research and years of experience

✓ For providers of cancer care all over the world

✓ Expert recommendations for cancer screening, diagnosis, and treatment

Free online at
NCCN.org/guidelines

NCCN Guidelines for Patients

✓ Present information from the NCCN Guidelines in an easy-to-learn format

✓ For people with cancer and those who support them

✓ Explain the cancer care options likely to have the best results

Free online at
NCCN.org/patientguidelines

These NCCN Guidelines for Patients are based on the NCCN Guidelines® for Bladder Cancer, Version 4.2021 — July 27, 2021.

NCCN Foundation seeks to support the millions of patients and their families affected by a cancer diagnosis by funding and distributing NCCN Guidelines for Patients. NCCN Foundation is also committed to advancing cancer treatment by funding the nation's promising doctors at the center of innovation in cancer research. For more details and the full library of patient and caregiver resources, visit NCCN.org/patients.

National Comprehensive Cancer Network (NCCN) / NCCN Foundation
3025 Chemical Road, Suite 100
Plymouth Meeting, PA 19462
215.690.0300

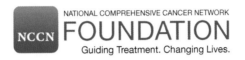

NCCN Guidelines for Patients are supported by funding from the NCCN Foundation®

With generous support from Wendy and David Rees

To make a gift or learn more, please visit NCCNFoundation.org/donate
or e-mail PatientGuidelines@NCCN.org.

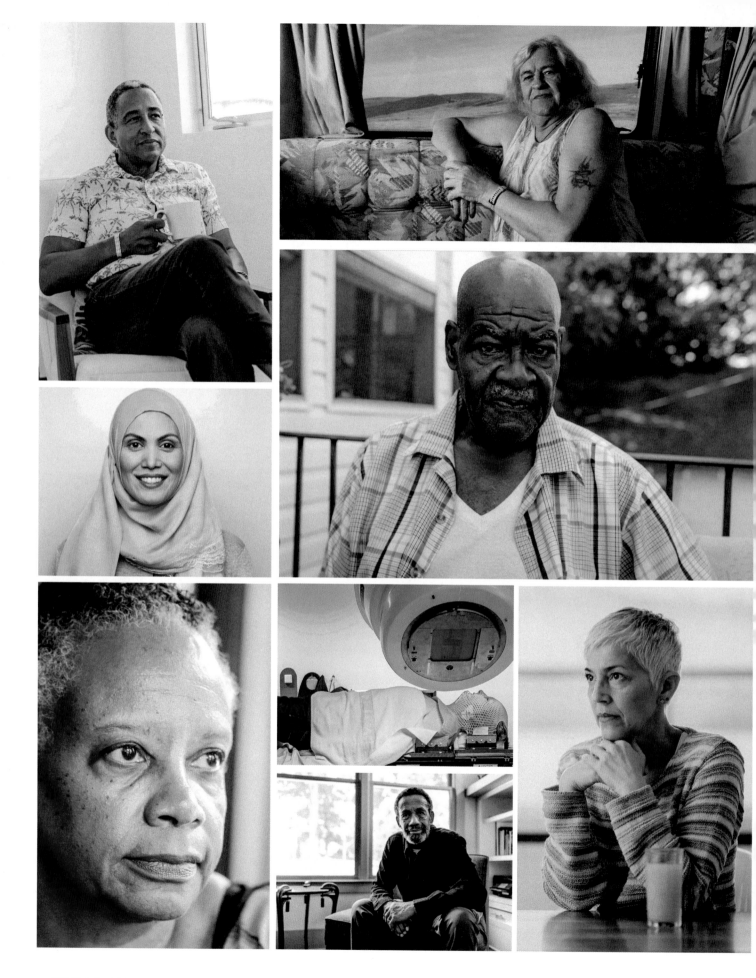

Contents

1
Bladder basics

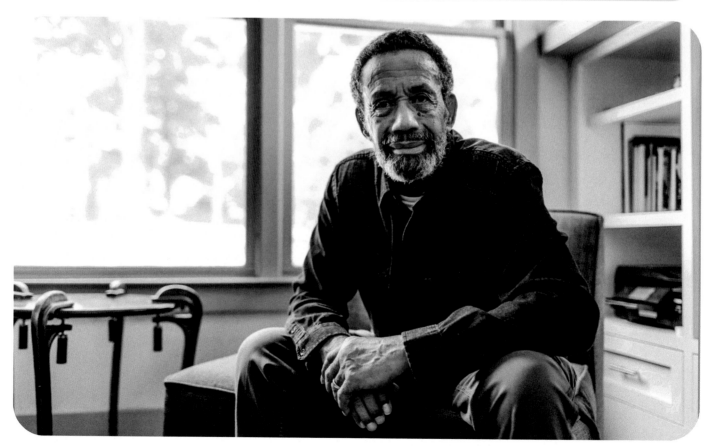

Urinary tract

The urinary tract, also referred to as the urinary system, includes 2 kidneys, 2 ureters, a bladder, and the urethra.

The urinary tract serves to:

> Eliminate waste from the body

> Regulate blood volume and blood pressure

> Control levels of electrolytes and metabolites (help regulate nerve and muscle function)

> Regulate blood pH (blood acidity or alkalinity)

Kidneys

The kidneys are organs shaped like beans. They are as big as the size of your fist. They are located just below your rib cage, one on each side of your spine. Every day, your kidneys filter about 120 to 150 quarts of blood to remove waste and balance fluids. This process produces about 1 to 2 quarts of urine per day.

Ureters

Ureters are thin tubes of muscle that connect your kidneys to your bladder. The ureters are about 8 to 10 inches long. Their job is to carry urine to the bladder. The muscles in the ureter walls tighten and relax to force urine away from the kidneys.

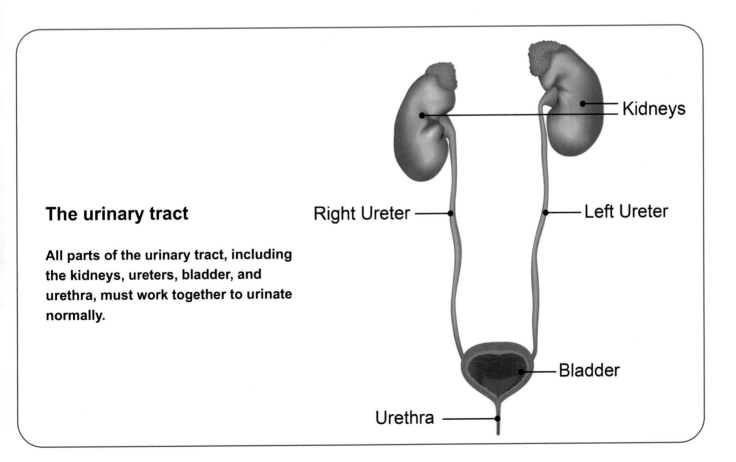

The urinary tract

All parts of the urinary tract, including the kidneys, ureters, bladder, and urethra, must work together to urinate normally.

Kidneys

Right Ureter —

Left Ureter

Bladder

Urethra —

Bladder

The bladder is a hollow, muscular, balloon-shaped organ that expands as it fills with urine. The bladder sits in your pelvis between your hip bones. A normal bladder acts like a reservoir (a place where urine collects). It can hold 1.5 to 2 cups of urine.

Urethra

The urethra is a tube located at the bottom of the bladder. This tube allows urine to exit the body during urination.

Bladder cancer

Bladder cancer is one of the most common cancers. It occurs mainly in people aged 55 years and over. Bladder cancer begins in the cells of the bladder. It most often affects the urothelial cells of the bladder. These cells form the lining of the entire urinary tract.

Most bladder cancers are diagnosed at an early stage, when the cancer is highly treatable. However, even after successful treatment you may have new occurrences or a recurrence of bladder cancer. People with bladder cancer typically need follow-up tests for years after treatment.

Symptoms

Symptoms of bladder cancer may include:

> Blood in urine (hematuria)

> Frequent urination

> Painful urination

> Back pain

> Urgency

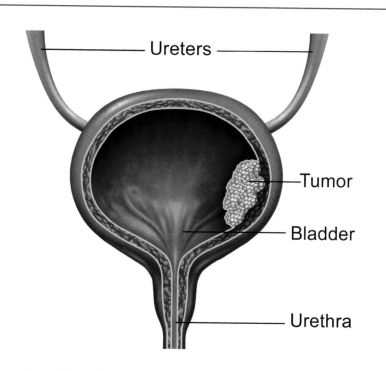

Bladder cancer

Bladder cancer is often described by how far it has spread into the muscle wall of the bladder.

Types of bladder cancer

Urothelial carcinoma

Urothelial carcinoma (transitional cell carcinoma) is the most common type of bladder cancer. Urothelial carcinoma starts in the urothelial cells. Urothelial cells are cells that line the inside of the bladder. Urothelial cells also line other parts of the urinary tract, such as the kidney, the ureters, and the urethra. People with bladder cancer may also have tumors in these places. It is important that these other areas are also checked for tumors.

Other types of bladder cancer

Although less common that urothelial carcinoma, there are other types of cancer that can start in the bladder.

They include:

> Adenocarcinoma

> Sarcoma

> Small cell carcinoma

> Squamous cell carcinoma

Adenocarcinoma

About 1 in 100 (or 1% of) bladder cancers are adenocarcinomas. Adenocarcinomas of the bladder have a higher likelihood of being invasive at diagnosis.

Sarcoma

Sarcomas are rare. They are found in the muscle cells of the bladder.

Small cell carcinoma

Small cell carcinoma starts in neuroendocrine (nerve-like) cells. Small cell carcinoma grows quickly.

Squamous cell carcinoma

About 5 percent (5%) of people with bladder cancer have squamous cell carcinoma. Squamous cell carcinomas have a higher chance of becoming invasive.

Where cancer is found

Bladder cancer is often described by how far it has spread into the wall (muscle) of the bladder:

Non-muscle invasive cancers

Non-muscle invasive cancers are found in the top layer of cells. They have not yet grown into the deeper cell layers. Stages 0 and 1 are non-muscle invasive. This is considered early bladder cancer. That means the tumor has not yet reached the deeper layer of muscle of the bladder wall surface.

Treatment goals for non-muscle invasive cancer are to:

> Reduce the risk of cancer recurrence after successful treatment

> Stop the cancer from metastasizing (spread to other areas of the body)

You may also see bladder cancer described as superficial. This term includes both non-invasive tumors as well as any invasive tumors that have not grown into the main muscle layer of the bladder.

Muscle invasive cancers

Muscle invasive cancers have grown into deeper layers of the bladder wall. These cancers are more likely to spread and are harder to treat. Muscle invasive cancers may be treated with surgery or radiation with chemotherapy to prevent the spread of the cancer cells far from the bladder.

Metastatic bladder cancer

Metastatic bladder cancer (stage 4) has spread to the abdominal wall, lymph nodes, and other areas far from the bladder. Stage 4 bladder cancer is generally not curable.

The goal for treatment is to help you live as comfortably as possible, for as long as possible.

Diagnosis

One of the first ways bladder cancer is diagnosed is by finding blood in the urine. The presence of blood can cause your urine to change color. If there is only a trace (small) amount of blood in the urine, hematuria may only be found during a urinalysis (urine test).

Some other ways bladder cancer is diagnosed:

➢ Frequent urination – people may have to urinate (pee) more often than usual

➢ Urgent urination – you may notice the need to urinate comes on quickly and is very intense.

➢ Painful urination – many people also experience pain while urinating. Bladder cancer can also cause pain in the low back and pelvis.

Early detection

One of the most common signs of bladder cancer is blood in the urine. Even if bleeding is occasional and short-lived and there is little or no pain associated with the bleeding, patients should not consider blood in the urine to be normal and should seek medical attention to determine the cause.

Risk factors

A risk factor is something that increases your chance of developing a disease. If you have been diagnosed with bladder cancer, your health care provider will consider a number of risk factors before identifying treatment options.

Risk factors associated with bladder cancer include:

➢ **Smoking:** Smoking is the greatest risk factor for bladder cancer.

➢ **Chemical exposure:** Some chemicals used in dyes, rubber, leather, printing materials, textiles, and paint products have been linked to an increased risk for bladder cancer.

➢ **Race:** Caucasians are twice (2x) as likely to develop bladder cancer.

➢ **Age:** The risk of bladder cancer increases as you age.

➢ **Gender:** Men are diagnosed with bladder cancer more often than women.

➢ **Personal history of bladder cancer:** Your risk increases if you or anyone in your family has had bladder cancer.

Key points

- The urinary tract, also referred to as the urinary system, includes 2 kidneys, 2 ureters, a bladder, and the urethra.

- Bladder cancer is one of the most common cancers. It occurs mainly in people aged 55 years and over.

- Most bladder cancers are diagnosed at an early stage, when the cancer is highly treatable.

- Urothelial carcinoma (transitional cell carcinoma) is the most common type of bladder cancer.

- One of the first ways bladder cancer is diagnosed is by finding blood in the urine.

2
Testing

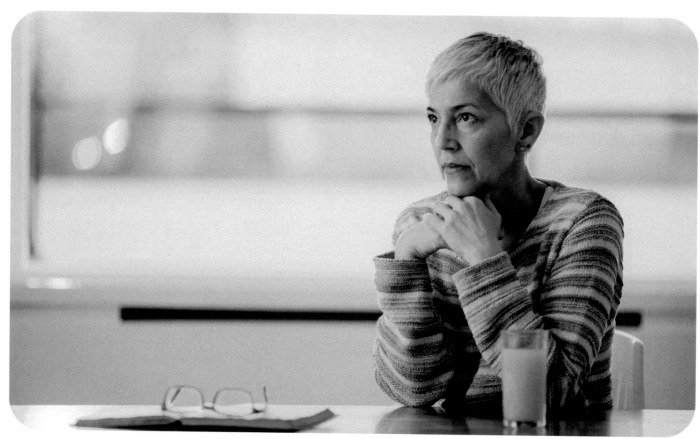

Treatment planning starts with testing. Accurate testing is needed to diagnose and treat bladder cancer. This chapter presents an overview of the tests you might receive and what to expect.

Test results

Results of your tests and possible imaging studies will determine your treatment plan. It is important to understand what these tests mean.

Keep these things in mind:

> Bring someone with you to doctor visits, if possible.

> Write down questions and take notes during appointments. Don't be afraid to ask your care team questions. Get to know your care team and let them get to know you.

> Get copies of blood tests, imaging results, and reports about the specific type of cancer you have.

> Organize your papers. Create files for insurance forms, medical records, and test results. You can do the same on your computer.

> Keep a list of contact information for everyone on your care team. Add it to your phone. Hang the list on your fridge or keep it in a place where someone can access it in an emergency.

A list of possible tests and procedures that you may receive are outlined in Guide 1.

Guide 1
Possible tests and procedures
Medical history and physical exam
Cystoscopy
Cytology
Abdominal or pelvic imaging
Screen for smoking

General health tests

Medical history

A medical history is a record of all health issues and treatments you have had in your life. Be prepared to list any illness or injury and when it happened. Bring a list of old and new medicines and any over-the-counter medicines, herbals, or supplements you take. Tell your doctor about any symptoms you have. A medical history will help determine which treatment is best for you.

Family history

Some cancers and other diseases can run in families. Your doctor will ask about the health history of family members who are blood relatives. This information is called a family history. Ask family members about their health issues like heart disease, cancer, and diabetes, and at what age they were diagnosed.

Physical exam

During a physical exam, your health care provider may:

> Check your temperature, blood pressure, pulse, and breathing rate

> Check your weight

> Listen to your lungs and heart

> Look in your eyes, ears, nose, and throat

> Feel and apply pressure to parts of your body to see if organs are of normal size, are soft or hard, or cause pain when touched. Tell your doctor if you feel pain.

> Feel for enlarged lymph nodes in your neck, underarm, and groin.

Ask questions and keep copies of your test results. Online patient portals are a great way to access test results.

Urine tests

Urine cytology

A urine cytology test uses a microscope to study your cells collected through urine. Your health care provider will be looking to see how the cells look and function. This test specifically looks for any cancer or precancerous conditions. You may receive a urine cytology test if you have blood in your urine (hematuria).

Cystoscopy

Cystoscopy is a procedure to see inside the bladder and urethra using a tool inserted through the urethra. Cystoscopy may be done in your doctor's office at the first visit, or it may be scheduled for a date in the near future. If your doctor sees any suspicious areas during the cystoscopy, more testing is needed.

Preparing for the procedure

You might be asked to:

> Take antibiotics. You may be asked to take antibiotics before and after the cystoscopy if you have trouble fighting off infections.

> Wait to empty your bladder. Wait to empty your bladder until your appointment. You may be asked to give a urine sample before the procedure.

Side effects

After a cystoscopy you may experience the following:

> Bleeding from your urethra, which can appear bright pink in your urine or on toilet tissue

> A burning sensation during urination

> More frequent urination for the next day or two

Speak to your doctor about what to expect after the procedure.

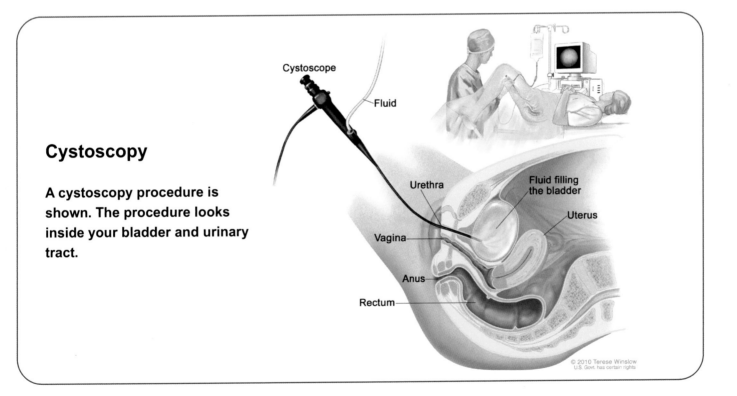

Cystoscopy

A cystoscopy procedure is shown. The procedure looks inside your bladder and urinary tract.

Cystoscope
Fluid
Urethra
Fluid filling the bladder
Uterus
Vagina
Anus
Rectum

© 2010 Terese Winslow
U.S. Govt. has certain rights

Imaging

Imaging tests are done to see if the cancer has spread to tissues, organs, and lymph nodes near the bladder, or to distant parts of your body. A biopsy may be used to evaluate any positive imaging tests.

CT scan

A computed tomography (CT or CAT) scan uses x-rays and computer technology to take pictures of the inside of the body. It takes many x-rays of the same body part from different angles. All the images are combined to make one detailed three-dimensional (3D) picture.

In most cases, you will be injected with a contrast solution. Contrast is used to improve the pictures of the inside of the body. Contrast materials help to enhance and improve the quality of the images. They are not dyes.

Talk to your health care providers if you have had allergic reactions to contrast in the past. This is important. You might be given medicines, such as Benadryl® and prednisone, to avoid the effects of those allergies. Contrast might not be used if you have a serious allergy or if your kidneys are not working well.

CT urography

A CT urogram is a test that uses x-rays to see how well your urinary tract is working. A urinary tract includes the kidneys, bladder, and ureters. X-rays allow your health care provider to produce multiple images to examine your bones, soft tissues, and blood vessels. During the test, you will be injected (in hand or arm) with an iodine contrast solution. The contrast helps to highlight your kidneys, ureters, and bladder.

Your health care provider may recommend a CT urogram if you are having symptoms such as pain in your side or back or have blood in your urine.

MRI

A magnetic resonance imaging (MRI) scan uses radio waves and powerful magnets to take pictures of the inside of the body. It does not use x-rays. Contrast might be used.

MR urography

A magnetic resonance (MR) urography test helps to find anything blocking the urinary tract, hematuria (blood in the urine), and birth defects (conditions developed before or at birth).

Renal ultrasound

A renal ultrasound uses sound waves to look at your kidneys, ureters, and bladder. The ultrasound is a painless test that produces black and white images to show the inside of your kidneys and other organs.

Retrograde ureteropyelography

A retrograde ureteropyelogram is an imaging test that uses x-rays to look at your ureters and kidneys. It is done with a rigid cystoscope in the operating room using dye injected into the ureter. The x-ray is used to evaluate how the dye flows. This test may also be used to find causes for blood in urine, such as a tumor, kidney stone, or blood clot.

Blood tests

Blood tests check for signs of disease and how well organs are working. They require a sample of your blood, which is removed through a needle placed into your vein.

Complete blood count

A complete blood count (CBC) measures the levels of red blood cells, white blood cells, and platelets in your blood. Your doctor will want to know if you have enough red blood cells to carry oxygen throughout your body, white blood cells to fight infection, and platelets to control bleeding.

Renal function testing

Renal function tests are used to evaluate functions of the kidneys. Your kidneys filter waste materials from the blood and get rid of them through your urine. Your kidneys also help control the levels of water and various essential minerals in your body. The tests measure levels of electrolytes and creatinine in the blood to determine the current health of your kidneys.

Create a medical binder

A medical binder or notebook is a great way to organize all of your records in one place.

- Make copies of blood tests, imaging results, and reports about your specific type of cancer. It will be helpful when getting a second opinion.

- Choose a binder that meets your needs. Consider a zipper pocket to include a pen, small calendar, and insurance cards.

- Create folders for insurance forms, medical records, and tests results. You can do the same on your computer.

- Use online patient portals to view your test results and other records. Download or print the records to add to your binder.

- Organize your binder in a way that works for you. Add a section for questions and to take notes.

- Bring your medical binder to appointments. You never know when you might need it!

Screen for smoking

Smokers are 3 times more likely than non-smokers to develop bladder cancer. While there is a lot of information about how smoking related toxins enter the body, there is little information about how these toxins exit the body. Toxins leave the body through the urinary tract. Chemicals from tobacco smoke or vaping are absorbed into the blood. Then they are passed from the kidneys into the urine and sit in the bladder until you urinate.

Your health care provider will ask you questions to find out about your tobacco use. Potential questions to expect are listed in Guide 2.

Many people believe vaping is safer than smoking. However, vaping (e-cigarettes) also leads to an increased risk for bladder cancer.

Guide 2
Potential questions to screen for smoking

Have you ever smoked cigarettes?

Do you currently smoke cigarettes or have you smoked in the last 30 days?

How much do you currently smoke or use nicotine (eg, cigarettes, pipes, cigars, e-cigarettes) per day?

What is the typical amount you smoked per day within the last 3 months?

How soon do you smoke after you wake up in the morning?

What is the longest period you have gone without smoking?

When was your last quit attempt?

Did you use anything to help you quit in the past? If so, what?

Why were previous quit attempts unsuccessful?

Are there other people in your house who use tobacco?

Key points

- Accurate testing is needed to diagnose and treat bladder cancer.

- Cystoscopy is a procedure used to see inside the bladder using a tool inserted through the urethra.

- A urine cytology test uses a microscope to study your cells collected through urine.

- Imaging tests are done to see if the cancer has spread to tissues, organs, and lymph nodes near the bladder, or to distant parts of your body.

- A computed tomography (CT) urogram is a test that uses x-rays to see how well your urinary tract is working and to evaluate the extent of the bladder cancer.

- A complete blood count (CBC) measures the levels of red blood cells, white blood cells, and platelets in your blood.

- Renal function tests are used to evaluate functions of the kidneys. Your kidneys filter waste materials from the blood and get rid of them through your urine.

3
Staging

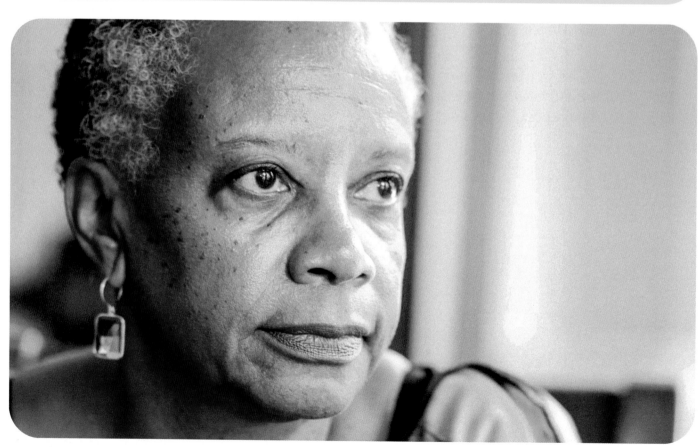

A cancer stage is a way to describe the extent of the cancer at the time you are first diagnosed. Cancer stages were created to determine how much cancer is in your body, where it is located, and what type you have. This is called staging.

TNM scores

The most commonly used staging system is the tumor, node, metastasis (TNM) staging system. In this system, the letters T, N, and M describe different areas of cancer growth. Based on imaging and biopsy results, your doctor will assign a score or number to each letter. The higher the number, the larger the tumor or the more the cancer has spread to lymph nodes or other organs. These scores will be combined to assign the cancer a stage.

A TNM example might look like this: T1N0M0 or T1, N0, M0.

> **T (tumor)** - Size of the main (primary) tumor

> **N (node)** - If cancer has spread to nearby (regional) lymph nodes

> **M (metastasis)** - If cancer has spread (metastasized) to distant parts of the body

T = Tumor

To describe how far a tumor has grown into the bladder wall, a number from 1 to 4 (and sometimes a letter) is used. The higher the number, the deeper the tumor has grown into the bladder wall. This is called the tumor stage.

The tumor stages for bladder cancer are described next.

> **Ta tumors** are called "papillary" tumors. Papillary tumors grow towards the inside of the bladder (called the lumen), where urine is held, rather than into the bladder wall. These tumors look like thin, finger-like growths. They are similar in appearance to broccoli stalks.

> **Tis tumors** refers to a flat area of fast-growing abnormal cells on the inside lining of the bladder. Tis is also called carcinoma in situ (CIS). These flat tumors are high-grade and need to be treated because they could become invasive bladder cancer.

> **T1 tumors** have grown into the connective tissue layer of the bladder wall, but not into the muscle layer. This is non-muscle invasive bladder cancer.

> **T2 tumors** have entered the muscle layer of the bladder wall. It may be only in the inner half of the muscle layer (a T2a tumor) or it may have invaded the outer half (a T2b tumor). This and later stages are muscle invasive bladder cancer.

> **T3 tumors** have grown all the way through the bladder wall and into the fatty tissue that surrounds the bladder.

> **T4 tumors** have invaded any of these nearby areas: the prostate, the glands that help produce semen (called the seminal vesicles), the uterus, the vagina, or the wall of the pelvis or abdomen.

N = Node

There are hundreds of lymph nodes in your body. They work as filters to help fight infection and to remove harmful things from the body. Doctors use a number from 0 to 3 to describe whether bladder cancer has spread to any lymph nodes in the pelvic region. The higher the number, the greater the extent of the lymph node involvement.

> **N0** means that cancer hasn't spread to any nearby lymph nodes.

> **N1** means that cancer has spread to only one lymph node in the pelvis.

> **N2** means that cancer has spread to more than one lymph node in the pelvis.

> **N3** means that cancer has spread to lymph nodes in the upper pelvic region, called the common iliac lymph nodes.

M = Metastasis

Cancer can spread far from the bladder. This process is called metastasis. Knowing whether the cancer has spread far from the bladder is an important part of choosing the best treatments. If your doctors don't know if the cancer has spread far, an MX is used.

> **M0** means that the cancer hasn't spread from your bladder.

> **M1** means that the cancer has spread to either distant lymph nodes (M1a) or to distant organs (M1b).

G = Grade

The next piece of information used to plan treatment for bladder cancer is called its grade. The grade is a rating of how fast your doctors think the cancer will grow and spread.

To figure out the grade, a sample of your tumor will be studied in a laboratory by a pathologist. The pathologist will compare the cancer cells to normal cells. The more different they look, the higher the grade and the faster the cancer is expected to spread.

> **LG** means that the cancer cells are low-grade (slow-growing).

> **HG** means that the cancer cells are high-grade (fast-growing).

Putting it all together

We just learned about these four key pieces of information your doctors need to know about your cancer:

> How far the tumor has grown through the bladder wall (the tumor stage)

> Whether any nearby lymph nodes are suspected of having cancer

> Whether the cancer has spread to lymph nodes or organs far from the bladder

> How fast the cancer is expected to grow (the tumor grade)

There are two types of stages for bladder cancer.

> **Clinical stage (c)** is the rating given before any treatment. It is based on imaging and biopsies before surgery.

> **Pathologic stage (p)** is based on the microscopic evaluation of the bladder and lymph nodes removed during surgery.

Stages of bladder cancer

There are 5 main stages of bladder cancer: 0, 1, 2, 3, and 4. Some of these stages are broken down into sub-groups. For the purposes of this book, bladder cancer will be separated based on whether it is non-muscle invasive disease or muscle invasive disease.

Non-muscle invasive stages

Non-muscle invasive cancer is confined to the bladder. It has not spread to lymph nodes or other parts of the body.

Stage 0a

One or more papillary tumors have formed on the inside lining of the bladder. This is the earliest stage of bladder cancer.

Stage 0is

There are flat areas of fast-growing abnormal cells called carcinoma in situ (CIS) on the inside lining of the bladder.

Stage 1

The tumor is invasive but has not reached the muscle layer of the wall.

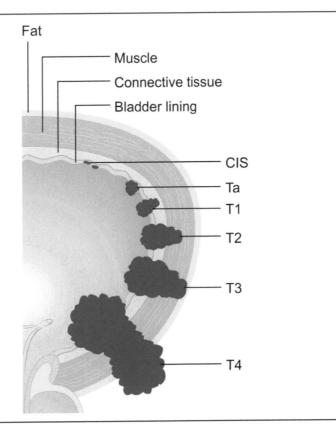

Stages of bladder cancer

There are 5 main stages of bladder cancer: 0, 1, 2, 3, and 4.

https://commons.wikimedia.org/wiki/File:Diagram_showing_the_T_stages_of_bladder_cancer_CRUK_372.svg

Fat

Muscle

Connective tissue

Bladder lining

CIS

Ta

T1

T2

T3

T4

Muscle invasive stages

Muscle invasive cancer has spread to lymph nodes or other parts of the body.

Stage 2

The tumor has invaded the muscle layer of the bladder wall. It may be only in the inner half of the muscle layer (a T2a tumor) or it may have invaded the outer half (a T2b tumor). Cancer has not spread to lymph nodes or organs far from the bladder.

Stage 3A

The tumor has not spread to lymph nodes or organs far from the bladder. The tumor may be any size. In this stage, cancer has spread beyond the bladder wall to surrounding tissues or organs.

Stage 3B

The tumor may be any size. Cancer has spread to multiple lymph nodes in the pelvis, or to lymph nodes in the upper pelvic region. Cancer has not spread to lymph nodes or organs far from the bladder.

Stage 4A

The tumor may be any size. The tumor has spread through the bladder wall to the pelvis, abdomen, or nearby lymph nodes.

Stage 4B

The tumor may be any size. Cancer has spread to lymph nodes and organs far from the bladder, like the bones, liver, or lungs. This is distant metastatic bladder cancer.

Key points

> Your cancer will be staged at the time of cancer diagnosis. This is called clinical staging.

> The stage is a rating to describe the size and how far it has spread. Your cancer stage will be used to determine which tests and treatments will help you receive the best outcome.

> The most commonly used staging system for bladder cancer is the TNM system.

> There are 5 overall stages of bladder cancer: 0, 1, 2, 3, and 4.

> For the purposes of this book, bladder cancer will be separated based on whether it is non-muscle invasive disease or muscle invasive disease.

> Stage 0 is non-invasive bladder cancer. This means that cancer has not grown beyond the second layer of the bladder wall.

> Muscle invasive bladder cancer has invaded the muscle layer of the bladder wall. This cancer can be stage 2, 3, or 4.

> Stage 4 is metastatic bladder cancer. This is cancer that has spread to distant sites in the body.

4
Treatment

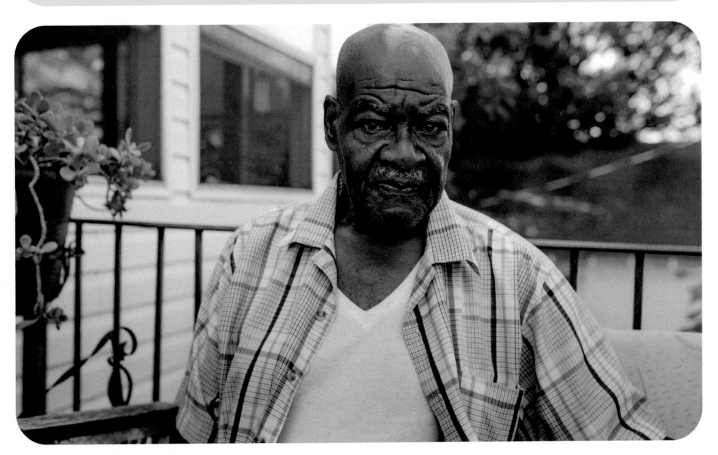

This chapter is a general overview of the types of treatment for bladder cancer and what to expect. Together, you and your doctor will choose a treatment plan that is right for you.

Treatment planning for bladder cancer is based on the extent, severity, and type of disease. Your age, ability to perform daily tasks, if you have other serious health issues, and drug availability and affordability all play a role in treatment decisions. Your wishes are always important.

TURBT

Transurethral resection of bladder tumor (TURBT) is a procedure that removes and examines tumors on the bladder wall.

Tumors are removed through the urethra without having to cut through the abdominal or pelvic skin. An instrument with a small cutting surface at one end is guided through the urethra and into the bladder to remove the tumor. This is done under general anesthesia in an operating room.

Goals of TURBT include:

> Confirm the bladder cancer diagnosis

> Determine how extensive the cancer is inside the bladder

> Remove all of the visible tumor

> Take a sample of the muscle layer of the bladder wall to see if the tumor has invaded muscle

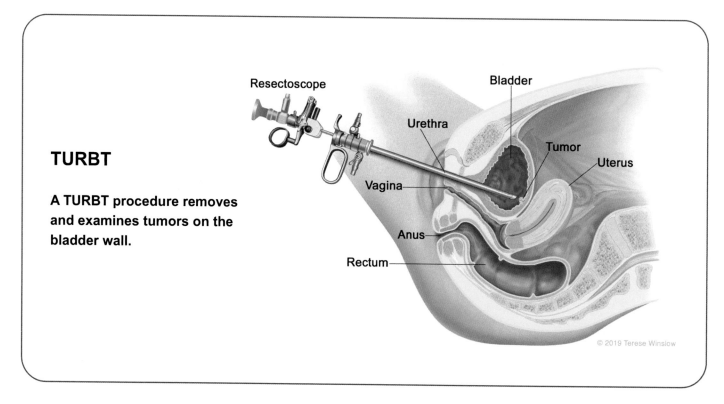

TURBT

A TURBT procedure removes and examines tumors on the bladder wall.

Resectoscope • Bladder • Urethra • Tumor • Uterus • Vagina • Anus • Rectum

© 2019 Terese Winslow

Radical cystectomy

Radical cystectomy is the most widely used surgery for muscle invasive bladder cancer. It involves removing the bladder, nearby lymph nodes, and other organs in the pelvis. Other nearby organs may also be removed.

Other organs may include:

> Prostate

> Seminal vesicles
(glands that help make semen)

> Part of the vas deferens (a tube that carries sperm away from the testicles)

> Proximal urethra (part of the urethra that goes through the prostate)

> The uterus

> The ovaries

> The fallopian tubes

> The urethra

> Part of the vagina

When your bladder is removed, you need a new way for urine to exit your body. This procedure is called a urinary diversion.

There are 3 types of urinary diversions:

> Ileal conduit

> Neobladder

> Continent urinary reservoir
(Indiana pouch)

Ileal conduit

After a radical cystectomy, you may receive an ileal conduit. In this procedure, your surgeon will create a new tube from a piece of intestine (ileum). This tube will allow your kidneys to drain. Your urine will now exit the body through a small opening called a stoma.

A small disposable bag attached to the outside of your abdomen collects urine when it comes out of the stoma. This is called an ostomy bag (or ostomy pouch). The bag stays attached to your body with the help of an adhesive part called a "wafer." The wafer sticks to the skin and acts as a watertight barrier.

Neobladder

The small intestine is repurposed to drain urine. The small bowel is utilized like a piece of fabric to create a bladder substitute. Like your original bladder, this substitute bladder is attached to the ureters at one end and your urethra at the other end.

This means that urine follows the same path out of the body it normally would if you still had your bladder. This approach does not use a stoma or require an ostomy bag, since urine leaves the body in the usual way.

Neobladders do not work in the same way as real bladders. It may be hard to control the flow of urine out of the body. In other words, urine might come out when you do not want it or expect it to, particularly during sleep. This is called urinary incontinence. Substitute bladders may be difficult to empty completely. Some people may need to have a catheter inserted through their urethra to help drain the urine from a substitute bladder.

Continent cutaneous urinary diversion

A continent cutaneous urinary diversion uses a segment of intestine to create a pouch to hold urine. The pouch has a channel for urine to pass through made from intestine that connects it to the wall of the abdomen. This is usually covered by a small bandage. Urine is drained through the pouch into a catheter. A tiny hole called a stoma is made in the abdominal wall at the location of the reservoir. A catheter must be inserted through the stoma, past the valve, and into the reservoir several times a day to drain the urine. Sometimes the stoma can be made in the belly button, making it much less noticeable.

A benefit to this type of urinary diversion is that an ostomy bag does not need to be worn on the outside of the body. This may be appealing to people with concerns about body image, and those who do not want to worry about an ostomy bag coming loose or leaking.

Partial cystectomy

A partial cystectomy is a surgical procedure to remove part of the bladder. It is not widely used for the treatment of bladder cancer. Fewer than 5 out of 100 people will meet the criteria for a partial (instead of a radical) cystectomy.

You may be eligible for a partial cystectomy if:

> The tumor is at the top of the bladder and there are no fast-growing (high-grade) cells in other areas of the bladder lining.

> The cancer is only in a small pouch sticking out from the bladder wall (called a diverticulum).

> You have other very serious health conditions that would prevent you from having a radical cystectomy.

Intravesical therapy

Intravesical therapy is the use of medicines placed directly into the bladder through a catheter. The medicines are slowly put into the bladder using a process called instillation. There are two main intravesical therapies used to treat bladder cancer:

> Intravesical bacillus Calmette-Guérin (BCG) therapy

> Intravesical chemotherapy

Intravesical BCG therapy

Intravesical bacillus Calmette-Guérin (BCG) therapy uses a liquid solution placed directly into your bladder. The solution contains a very weak version of a bacterium (germ). The solution has been found to jumpstart your immune system and cause it to attack cancer cells inside the bladder.

Common side effects include:

> Difficulty or pain when urinating

> Urine leakage

> Bladder or groin pain

> Particles in your urine (not blood)

> Fever

> Chills

Talk to your health care provider about any side effects you experience. They may be able to help lessen the effects.

Intravesical BCG therapy is often given in two ways:

> Induction (first 6-week) treatment

> Maintenance treatment

Induction treatment
Primary treatment is one that is given first and expected to work best. BCG therapy is often used as the first treatment therapy for people with non-muscle invasive bladder cancer. Given after surgery (TURBT), it has shown to lower the chance of recurrence (cancer coming back), or getting worse (muscle invasive).

Intravesical BCG has been shown to be better at preventing the return of cancer than TURBT alone or TURBT with chemotherapy. BCG is usually started 3 to 4 weeks after TURBT. It is given once a week for 6 weeks, followed by a rest period of 4 to 6 weeks. You should have a full re-evaluation 12 weeks after the date you start treatment.

Maintenance treatment
Maintenance treatment is therapy provided to keep cancer cells from coming back. If you were successfully treated with BCG therapy, you may be asked to continue to reduce the risk of recurrence (cancer returning). Most people receive maintenance intravesical BCG therapy for anywhere between 1 to 3 years. Length of therapy depends on the person's risk of recurrence.

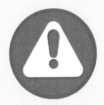

BCG shortage

There is an ongoing shortage of BCG in the United States. Because of this, its use is often limited to treating individuals with high-risk non-muscle invasive bladder cancer (cT1 high grade or CIS).

For people who do not receive BCG, intravesical (local) chemotherapy treatment may be used as an alternative.

Other options your health care provider may suggest include:

• Using a reduced dose of BCG

• Going straight to surgery (for those at high risk of the cancer returning after treatment)

• Joining a clinical trial

Intravesical (local) chemotherapy

Intravesical (local) chemotherapy is given to reduce the risk of the cancer recurrence, or to slow your cancer's growth to a higher stage. This type of chemotherapy is placed directly into the bladder through a catheter. These chemotherapy drugs are used to kill actively growing cancer cells.

Typical drugs for intravesical chemotherapy include gemcitabine, mitomycin C, and valrubicin.

> Gemcitabine (Gemzar®, Infugem™) is the preferred drug. It has fewer side effects than mitomycin and is less likely to be absorbed into the blood.

> Mitomycin is used most often for superficial tumors.

> Valrubicin (Valstar®) may be used in certain circumstances.

The main side effects of intravesical therapy are irritation and burning in the bladder, and blood in the urine.

Immediately after TURBT

When given after TURBT, intravesical chemotherapy is shown to lower the risk of recurrence. The one-time dose is to be given within 24 hours of surgery.

Primary treatment

Intravesical chemotherapy is an option for primary treatment if BCG therapy is not available. Treatment usually begins 3 to 4 weeks after TURBT. You can expect to receive treatments once a week for 6 weeks.

Systemic therapy

A cancer treatment that affects the whole body is called systemic therapy. The most common type of systemic therapy is chemotherapy. Chemotherapy and other types of systemic therapy are described next.

Chemotherapy

Chemotherapy is treatment with drugs to kill cancer cells. Most chemotherapy drugs are liquids that are slowly injected into a vein. This process is called infusion. The drugs travel in your bloodstream to treat cancer throughout your body. Chemotherapy may also harm healthy cells. Speak to your health care provider about any potential side effects from your chemotherapy treatment.

Targeted therapy

Targeted therapy is a cancer treatment that can target and attack specific types of cancer cells. This type of cancer treatment is often used for people with specific gene mutations. If you do not have the mutation that the medicine "targets," treatment is unlikely to help you. For example, erdafitinib (Balversa™) is a targeted therapy used for bladder cancer that targets mutations of specific genes called the *FGFR2* and *FGFR3* genes.

Immunotherapy

Immunotherapy is a cancer treatment that increases the activity of your body's immune system. By doing so, it can improve your body's ability to find and destroy cancer cells. Immunotherapy medicines called checkpoint inhibitors (drugs that block proteins called checkpoints) are used to treat bladder and other cancers.

Radiation therapy

Radiation therapy specific to bladder cancer is called external beam radiation therapy (EBRT). In EBRT, a large machine aims radiation at the tumor area. Radiation therapy (RT) uses radiation from electrons, photons, x-rays, protons, gamma rays, and other sources to kill cancer cells and shrink tumors. RT can be given alone or with other treatments.

Chemoradiotherapy

Chemotherapy and radiation therapy are used together to try to kill the cancer. When given together, they work better than they do alone. Like any treatment, chemoradiation has been shown to work better for certain people than for others. Speak to your health care provider about this treatment option.

> External beam radiation therapy is used to treat bladder cancer. A source outside the body focuses radiation on the cancer.

Bring someone to appointments

Many people miss things discussed in doctor's appointments. Bring someone whom you trust to listen and ask questions.

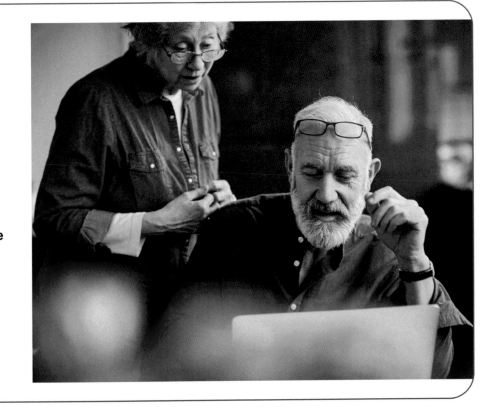

Clinical trials

A clinical trial is a type of medical research study. After being developed and tested in a laboratory, potential new ways of fighting cancer need to be studied in people. If found to be safe and effective in a clinical trial, a drug, device, or treatment approach may be approved by the U.S. Food and Drug Administration (FDA).

Everyone with cancer should carefully consider all of the treatment options available for their cancer type, including standard treatments and clinical trials. Talk to your doctor about whether a clinical trial may make sense for you.

Phases

Most cancer clinical trials focus on treatment. Treatment trials are done in phases.

> **Phase 1** trials study the safety and side effects of an investigational drug or treatment approach.

> **Phase 2** trials study how well the drug or approach works against a specific type of cancer.

> **Phase 3** trials test the drug or approach against a standard treatment. If the results are good, it may be approved by the FDA.

> **Phase 4** trials study the long-term safety and benefit of an FDA-approved treatment.

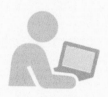

Finding a clinical trial

In the United States

NCCN Cancer Centers
NCCN.org/cancercenters

The National Cancer Institute (NCI)
cancer.gov/about-cancer/treatment/clinical-trials/search

Worldwide

The U.S. National Library of Medicine (NLM)
clinicaltrials.gov/

Need help finding a clinical trial?
NCI's Cancer Information Service (CIS)
1.800.4.CANCER (1.800.422.6237)
cancer.gov/contact

Who can enroll?

Every clinical trial has rules for joining, called eligibility criteria. The rules may be about age, cancer type and stage, treatment history, or general health. These requirements ensure that participants are alike in specific ways.

Informed consent

Clinical trials are managed by a group of experts called a research team. The research team will review the study with you in detail, including its purpose and the risks and benefits of joining. All of this information is also provided in an informed consent form. Read the form carefully and ask questions before signing it. Take time to discuss with family, friends, or others whom you trust. Keep in mind that you can leave and seek treatment outside of the clinical trial at any time.

Start the conversation

Don't wait for your doctor to bring up clinical trials. Start the conversation and learn about all of your treatment options. If you find a study that you may be eligible for, ask your treatment team if you meet the requirements. Try not to be discouraged if you cannot join. New clinical trials are always becoming available.

Frequently asked questions

There are many myths and misconceptions surrounding clinical trials. The possible benefits and risks are not well understood by many with cancer.

Will I get a placebo?

Placebos (inactive versions of real medicine) are almost never used alone in cancer clinical trials. It is common to receive either a placebo with standard treatment, or a new drug with standard treatment. You will be informed, verbally and in writing, if a placebo is part of a clinical trial before you are enrolled.

Do I have to pay to be in a clinical trial?

Rarely. It depends on the study, your health insurance, and the state in which you live. Your treatment team and the research team can help determine if you are responsible for any costs.

Key points

- Treatment options will depend on the stage of your cancer and your preferences.

- Transurethral resection of bladder tumor (TURBT) is a procedure that removes and examines tumors on the bladder wall.

- Radical cystectomy is the most widely used surgery for muscle invasive bladder cancer. It involves removing the bladder, nearby lymph nodes, and other organs in the pelvis.

- A partial cystectomy is a surgical procedure to remove part of the bladder. It is not widely used for the treatment of bladder cancer.

- Intravesical therapy is the use of medicines placed directly into the bladder through a catheter. The medicines are slowly put into the bladder using a process called instillation.

- A cancer treatment that affects the whole body is called systemic therapy. The most common type of systemic therapy is chemotherapy.

- Radiation therapy specific to bladder cancer is called external beam radiation therapy (EBRT). In EBRT, a large machine aims radiation at the tumor area.

- Everyone with cancer should carefully consider all of the treatment options available for their cancer type, including standard treatments and clinical trials. Talk to your doctor about whether a clinical trial may make sense for you.

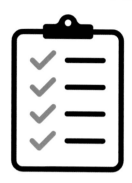

We want your feedback!

Our goal is to provide helpful and easy-to-understand information on cancer.

Take our survey to let us know what we got right and what we could do better:

NCCN.org/patients/feedback

5
Non-muscle invasive

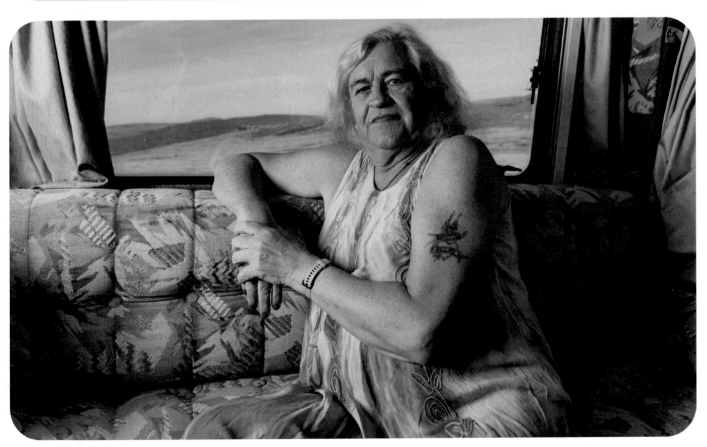

Non-muscle invasive bladder cancer refers to a tumor that has not yet grown into the muscle layer of the bladder wall. Stage 0 and stage 1 bladder cancers are non-muscle invasive. Treatment focuses on reducing the chance of recurrence and preventing the cancer from moving to a more advanced stage.

Stage 0

In stage 0 bladder cancer, the cancer is found only on the surface of the inner lining of the bladder.

Stage 0 is divided into two types depending on the type of tumor:

> **Stage 0a** - also called noninvasive papillary carcinoma, describes slender, finger-like projections from the inner surface of the bladder.

> **Stage 0is** - also called carcinoma in situ, describes a flat tumor on the tissue lining on the inside of the bladder.

Stage 0 bladder cancer is treated with a transurethral resection for bladder tumor (TURBT). You will then receive a follow-up appointment without further treatment or treatment with intravesical bacillus Calmette-Guérin (BCG) therapy.

Stage 1

In stage 1 bladder cancer, the tumor has grown into the bladder wall. Many of these tumors are high-grade (fast-growing) and likely to come back after treatment. If the disease is high grade, you may require a second TURBT to confirm the staging and remove any tumor left behind. For this reason, you may need to have a second TURBT.

Treatment for stage 1 is dependent on whether a second TURBT is done and if the test found cancer.

Cancer found during second TURBT
If you have a second TURBT, further treatment will depend on whether cancer cells are found and how deep they are in the bladder wall.

If cancer is found during the second TURBT, there are two treatment options:

> Intravesical BCG therapy

> Radical cystectomy (surgery)

Most people can be safely and effectively treated with intravesical BCG therapy. If BCG therapy is used, you may also receive maintenance BCG therapy. Maintenance therapy is given to help keep cancer from coming back after primary treatment. Maintenance BCG therapy may continue for years.

People at higher risk, however, will need surgery to remove the bladder (radical cystectomy). For example, surgery may be needed if the second TURBT found that a high-grade tumor has grown into the muscle layer of the bladder wall. For people who are not candidates for surgery, having chemoradiation (chemo and radiation together) is an option.

No cancer found during second TURBT

There are 2 treatment options if no cancer is found during the second TURBT:

> Intravesical BCG therapy

> Intravesical (local) chemotherapy

BCG therapy is the preferred treatment option. If you receive BCG therapy, you may be asked to continue with maintenance BCG therapy to prevent recurrence.

If you receive local chemotherapy, expect to be treated with gemcitabine or mitomycin. Gemcitabine is the preferred treatment drug.

Straight to surgery (no second TURBT)

Standard treatment for stage 1 bladder cancer is often a second TURBT. However, those with fast-growing tumors may need to have a radical cystectomy (surgery to remove the bladder).

The bladder may need to be removed due to the following:

> There is more than one tumor in the same area or multiple areas of the bladder

> The tumor is a rare subtype of bladder cancer that usually leads to poor outcomes

> There are tumor cells in the blood or lymph vessels outside of the main tumor (called lymphovascular invasion)

Follow-up care

When you have finished treatment, the next phase of cancer care will begin. This is the surveillance phase. During this time, it is important to have testing to monitor for your cancer returning. The specific tests you should have—and how often you should have them—are guided by your risk of cancer recurrence. It is important to keep any follow-up appointments with health care providers or for testing.

Speak to your doctor about who will lead your follow-up care. Some people continue to see their oncologist while others go back to their primary care provider.

Recurrence

Follow-up cystoscopy found cancer

One of the tests you will receive after completing treatment for bladder cancer is a cystoscopy. A cystoscopy is a procedure to see inside the bladder and other organs of the urinary tract using a tool inserted through the urethra. If cystoscopy results indicate cancer is present, you will likely have another TURBT.

Like the first TURBT, you should also have a single dose of local (intravesical) chemotherapy within 24 hours of the procedure. Treatment after the second TURBT depends on how far the tumor has grown through the bladder wall, and whether the tumor is slow- or fast-growing.

The treatment options include:

> **Intravesical (local) chemotherapy.** In order to decide if this is the best treatment option for you, your doctor will consider the risk of the cancer returning and the risk of it progressing to muscle invasive disease.

> **Radical cystectomy.** (surgery)

> **Chemoradiation.** This is an option if you are not a candidate for surgery and the tumor is small.

> **Clinical trial**

After treatment, you should have a follow-up visit in 3 months.

Suspicious follow-up urine cytology

More testing is needed if follow-up urine cytology (testing) finds that cancer may have returned. Further testing will look for cancer in other areas such as the prostate and upper urinary tract.

Tests may include:

> Biopsies of the bladder, prostate, and/or upper urinary tract

> Urine cytology of the upper urinary tract

> Ureteroscopy, a test that examines the lining of your kidneys and ureters

If the biopsy of the bladder finds cancer, BCG therapy is recommended. If BCG therapy works and cancer is no longer found, you may continue to receive BCG therapy to prevent recurrence.

If BCG therapy does not work, treatment options include:

> Radical cystectomy (surgery)

> Other intravesical therapies

> Chemoradiation (if you are not a candidate for surgery)

> Clinical trial

Next steps for test results:

> If positive biopsy for prostate cancer, treatment of the prostate is needed.

> If positive urine cytology test, treatment of the upper urinary tract is needed.

> If all of the tests are negative, you should have a follow-up visit in 3 months. Other visits will be spaced farther apart.

Cancer returned after intravesical therapy

If cancer is found after you have received 2 rounds of intravesical therapy, you will receive another form of treatment. Intravesical therapy is recommended to only be given 2 times (2x) back-to-back. Therefore, you can expect to have a transurethral resection of bladder tumor (TURBT) to help determine the extent of the cancer.

You will receive a single dose of intravesical (local) chemotherapy within 24 hours of the TURBT procedure. The most common medicines used are gemcitabine (preferred) and mitomycin C. If no remaining cancer cells are found, people who were on BCG therapy should continue to have maintenance BCG. Otherwise, no further treatment is needed.

If the TURBT finds cancer, the treatment you receive next depends on how far the tumor has grown through the bladder wall and whether the tumor is slow- or fast-growing.

Treatment options include:

> Other intravesical therapy

> Radical cystectomy (surgery) - Preferred for fast-growing (high-grade) T1 tumors

> Chemoradiation (if you are not a candidate for surgery)

> Clinical trial

Key points

> Non-muscle invasive bladder cancer refers to a tumor that has not yet grown into the muscle layer of the bladder wall.

> Stage 0 and stage 1 bladder cancers are non-muscle invasive.

> In stage 0 bladder cancer, the cancer is found only on the surface of the inner lining of the bladder. This stage is also referred to as in situ.

> Most people can be safely and effectively treated with intravesical BCG therapy. If BCG therapy is used, you may also receive maintenance BCG therapy.

> If you receive local chemotherapy, expect to be treated with gemcitabine or mitomycin. Gemcitabine is the preferred treatment drug.

6
Muscle invasive

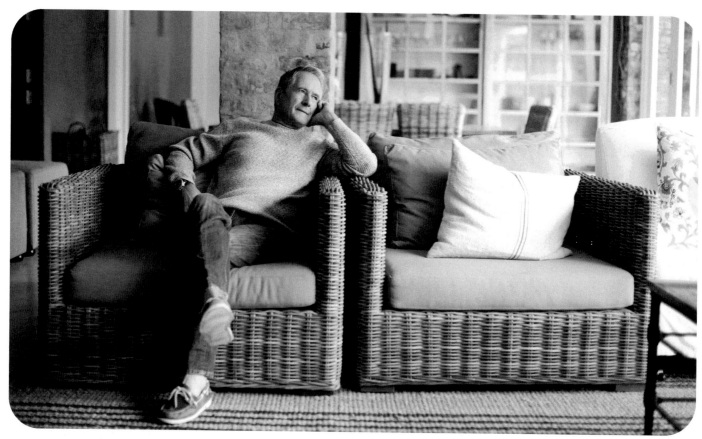

If the tumor grows large enough to reach the thick layer of muscle in the bladder wall, it is called muscle invasive bladder cancer. Bladder cancers that are staged at 2 or higher are considered muscle invasive. This is often treated with surgery or chemoradiation therapy.

Stage 2

Stage 2 bladder cancer describes a tumor that has grown less than halfway through the muscle wall of the bladder (a T2a tumor) or more than halfway through (a T2b tumor). In both instances, the cancer has not yet spread to lymph nodes or organs far from the bladder.

If you have stage 2 bladder cancer, you may receive further testing before treatment begins.

Testing may include:

> Abdominal pelvic CT or MRI

> Chest imaging

> Bone scan (if potential for bone metastases)

> Glomerular filtration rate (GRF) – The purpose of this test is to see if you can tolerate a chemotherapy drug called cisplatin.

Treatment for stage 2 bladder cancer is based on whether you are able to receive surgery to remove the bladder.

Cystectomy

A partial cystectomy removes part of the bladder. A radical cystectomy removes the entire bladder. It is the most common surgery for muscle invasive bladder cancer.

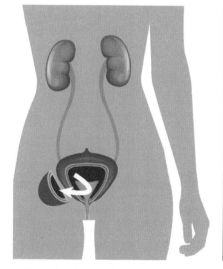
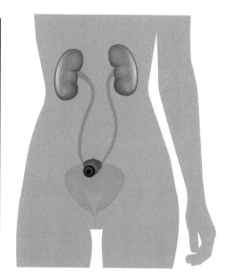

Partial Cystecomy   Radical Cystecomy

Cystectomy candidates

If you are able to receive a cystectomy, you can expect to receive one of the following treatment options found in Guide 3.

Chemotherapy and radical cystectomy

Before you receive surgery (radical cystectomy), you will receive a cisplatin-based chemotherapy. Cisplatin is a chemotherapy drug that has been shown to be most effective at treating bladder cancer. However, cisplatin may be too harsh for those whose liver and kidneys do not work well. Speak to your health care provider about any concerns you may have.

After finishing chemotherapy, you will receive a radical cystectomy. A radical cystectomy is the gold-standard surgery for muscle invasive bladder cancer. A radical cystectomy involves removing the bladder and prostate in men or the bladder and uterus in women.

Chemotherapy and partial cystectomy

A small number of people (about 5 out of 100) may be able to have a partial cystectomy. A partial cystectomy removes part of the bladder. During a partial cystectomy, an incision is made in the lower abdomen to expose your bladder. Nearby lymph nodes may be removed to be checked for cancer cells (to see if the cancer has spread). The part of the bladder with cancer is removed as well as an area (margin) of healthy tissue. The remaining bladder is closed with stitches.

You may be eligible for a partial cystectomy if:

> The tumor is at the top of the bladder and there are no fast-growing (high-grade) cells in other areas of the bladder lining

> The cancer is only in a small pouch sticking out from the bladder wall (called a diverticulum)

Guide 3 Treatment options: Stage 2 cystectomy candidates	
Primary treatment	• Neoadjuvant cisplatin-based chemotherapy and radical cystectomy • Neoadjuvant cisplatin-based chemotherapy and partial cystectomy • Cystectomy • Bladder preservation with chemoradiotherapy
Adjuvant treatment	• Adjuvant cisplatin-based chemotherapy (if no neoadjuvant treatment) • Adjuvant RT • Observation • Intravesical BCG • Surgical consolidation

> - You have other very serious health conditions that would prevent you from having a radical cystectomy

You will be treated before the surgery with a cisplatin-based chemotherapy.

Surgery alone

For those who are unable to have cisplatin-based chemotherapy, you will receive a cystectomy only. You may not be able to have cisplatin if you have hearing loss, nerve damage, kidney problems, or if you are not able to do most daily activities. If you cannot have cisplatin, you should not have any chemotherapy before surgery.

Adjuvant treatment after surgery

After surgery, you may receive treatment based on risk for cancer recurrence. This is called adjuvant therapy. Treatment options include cisplatin-based chemotherapy (if you did not receive it before surgery) or radiation therapy (RT).

Reasons you may have radiation therapy include:

> - The tumor was larger than expected
> - The surgeon found cancer in lymph nodes
> - The tumor started growing into the fatty tissue that surrounds the bladder

Bladder preservation with chemoradiotherapy

As an alternative to surgery, you may be eligible for trimodality therapy (TMT). TMT tries to preserve your bladder by using a transurethral resection of bladder tumor (TURBT) followed by chemoradiation therapy (CRT). TURBT is a procedure that removes and examines tumors on the bladder wall. CRT is a combination of chemotherapy and radiation therapy. The combination of therapies have been found to be more effective in preventing cancer recurrence.

You can expect to be tested for cancer recurrence 2 to 3 months after completing treatment. If there is no tumor present, you will be observed for any new signs or symptoms.

If a tumor is found, you may be treated with any of the following:

> - Intravesical BCG
> - Surgical consolidation

You may also be treated for metastatic disease. Speak with your health care provider regarding the best option for you.

Not a candidate for cystectomy

There are several reasons why you may not be able to have a radical cystectomy. If you have other serious health problems or are not physically able to do many day-to-day activities, surgery may not be an option for you. You also may not want surgery. Speak to your doctor about your options.

There are 3 treatment options that do not involve removing the bladder. They include:

> Chemoradiotherapy (preferred)

> Radiation therapy (RT)

> Transurethral resection of bladder tumor (TURBT)

Chemoradiotherapy

In chemoradiotherapy, chemotherapy and radiation therapy are used together to try to kill the cancer. When given together, they work better than they do alone. This option allows you to keep your bladder. Like any treatment, chemoradiation has been shown to work better for certain people than for others. Speak to your health care provider about this option for treatment.

Radiation therapy alone

Radiation therapy alone is for those who cannot have surgery or chemotherapy. Radiation therapy uses high-energy beams focused on a certain area to kill cancer cells.

TURBT

If you cannot have (or do not want) surgery to remove your bladder, having another TURBT is an option for people with stage 2 bladder cancer.

Adjuvant treatment

Adjuvant treatment refers to treatment provided after the first-line treatment is used. Before you receive adjuvant treatment, you will be assessed within 2 to 3 months after the primary treatment is completed. If no tumors are present at this time, you will be observed for any new signs or symptoms.

If a tumor is found, you may receive one of the following options:

> Systemic therapy

> Concurrent chemoradiotherapy

> RT

> TURBT with or without intravesical therapy

> Best supportive care

Follow-up

The size of the tumor should be checked within 2 to 3 months after you have completed treatment. If the tumor is gone, you can begin follow-up care and monitoring for the return of cancer. If you responded well to BCG therapy during treatment, you should have maintenance BCG therapy.

If the tumor is still there, there are 4 options:

> Chemotherapy

> Chemoradiation (only if you have not already had any radiation therapy)

> TURBT to try to relieve symptoms caused by the tumor

> Supportive care

Stage 3A

Stage 3 bladder cancer describes a tumor that has spread beyond the bladder wall to surrounding tissue and/or organs, and possibly to lymph nodes. The tumor has not spread to distant organs.

If you have stage 3A bladder cancer, you may receive further testing before treatment begins.

Testing may include:

> Abdominal pelvic CT or MRI

> Chest imaging

> Bone scan (if potential for bone metastases)

> Glomerular filtration rate (GRF) – the purpose of this test is to see if you can tolerate a chemotherapy drug called cisplatin.

Primary treatment for stage 3A bladder cancer is broken up by whether you are able to receive surgery to remove the bladder.

Cystectomy candidates

The following are options for those where a cystectomy is possible.

Chemotherapy and radical cystectomy

Before you receive surgery (radical cystectomy), you will receive a cisplatin-based chemotherapy. Cisplatin is a chemotherapy drug that has been shown to be most effective at treating bladder cancer. However, cisplatin may be too harsh for those whose liver and kidneys do not work well. Speak to your health care provider about any concerns you may have.

> Best supportive care refers to programs and services to help meet the needs and improve the quality of life of people living with cancer and their caregivers.

After finishing chemotherapy, you will receive a radical cystectomy. A radical cystectomy is the gold-standard surgery for muscle invasive bladder cancer. A radical cystectomy involves removing the bladder and prostate or bladder and uterus.

Surgery alone

For those who are unable to have cisplatin-based chemotherapy, you will receive a cystectomy only. You may not be able to have cisplatin if you have hearing loss, nerve damage, kidney problems, or if you are not able to do most activities.

Adjuvant treatment

Adjuvant treatment refers to treatment provided after surgery. If you received chemotherapy and surgery or just surgery as primary treatment, you may receive an adjuvant treatment to prevent recurrence. Treatment options include cisplatin-based chemotherapy (if not used before) or radiation therapy (for those who are high-risk).

Bladder preservation with chemoradiotherapy

As an alternative to surgery, you may be eligible for trimodality therapy (TMT). TMT tries to preserve your bladder by using a transurethral resection of bladder tumor (TURBT) followed by chemoradiation therapy (CRT). TURBT is a procedure that removes and examines tumors on the bladder wall. CRT is a combination of chemotherapy and radiation therapy.

You can expect to be tested for cancer recurrence 2 to 3 months after completing treatment. If there is no tumor present, you will be observed for any new signs or symptoms.

If a tumor is found, you will be treated with any of the following:

> Intravesical BCG (if tumor is small enough)

> Surgical consolidation (if limited to one organ)

You may also be treated as having metastatic disease. Speak with your health care provider regarding the best option for you.

Not a candidate for cystectomy

If you have other serious health problems or are not physically able to do many day-to-day activities, surgery may not be an option for you.

If surgery is not an option for you, you will be treated with 2 options:

> Chemoradiotherapy (preferred)

> Radiation therapy alone (RT)

Chemoradiotherapy

This option allows you to keep your bladder. Chemotherapy and radiation therapy are used together to try to kill the cancer. When given together, they work better than they do alone. Like any treatment, chemoradiation has been shown to work better for certain people than for others. Speak to your health care provider about this option for treatment.

Radiation therapy

This treatment option is only for people who cannot have surgery or chemotherapy. Radiation therapy uses high-energy beams focused on a certain area to kill cancer cells.

You can expect to be tested for cancer recurrence 2 to 3 months after completing treatment. If there is no tumor present, you will be observed for any new signs or symptoms.

If a tumor is found, you will be treated with any of the following:

> Systemic therapy

> TURBT with or without intravesical therapy

> Best supportive care

Stage 3B

Stage 3 bladder cancer has spread to multiple lymph nodes in the pelvis, or to lymph nodes in the upper pelvic region.

If you have stage 3B bladder cancer, you may receive further testing before treatment begins.

Testing may include:

> Abdominal pelvic CT or MRI

> Chest imaging

> Bone scan (if potential for bone metastases)

> Glomerular filtration rate (GRF) – to help determine eligibility for treatment with cisplatin

> Molecular or genomic testing – consider to determine family history

Primary treatment for stage 3B bladder cancer is broken up by 2 different therapy options, systemic therapy and chemoradiotherapy.

Order of treatments

Most people with bladder cancer will receive more than one type of treatment. Next is an overview of the order of treatments and what they do.

- **Neoadjuvant (before)** treatment is given to shrink the tumor before primary treatment (surgery).

- **Primary treatment** is the main treatment given to rid the body of cancer. Surgery is usually the main treatment for bladder cancer.

- **Adjuvant (after) treatment** is given after primary treatment to rid the body of any cancer cells left behind from surgery. It is also used when the risk of cancer returning (recurrence) is felt to be high.

- **First-line treatment** is the first set of treatments given.

- **Second-line treatment** is the next set of treatments given after the first treatment has failed.

Talk to your doctor about your treatment plan and what it means for your stage of bladder cancer.

Systemic therapy

Systemic therapy is used to shrink the tumor as much as possible. If the treatment is successful, the tumor stage and size may go down. For this reason, you may hear it be called "downstaging" systemic therapy. Treatment with systemic therapy depends on whether you can tolerate chemotherapy with the drug cisplatin. For a list of drugs used for systemic therapy, see Guide 4.

Within 2 to 3 months after treatment with systemic therapy, you will be tested to determine if the cancer responded to treatment. Tests may include CT imaging of the chest, abdomen, and/or pelvis with contrast.

You may have any of the following responses:

> Complete response

> Partial response

> Disease progression

Complete response

If you had a complete response to systemic therapy, having no further treatment is an option. A complete response is defined as no remaining signs of cancer in response to treatment. This does not always mean the cancer has been cured. In the case of a complete response, you would start monitoring for the return of cancer.

Another option is to have more treatment to kill any remaining cancer cells. This is called consolidation therapy. The goal of consolidation therapy is to help "lock in" your good results from treatment with systemic therapy. Consolidation therapy is like a "final sweep" for leftover cancer cells still in the body.

Consolidation treatments may include:

> Surgery (radical cystectomy)

> Chemoradiotherapy

Guide 4 Systemic therapy options: Stage 4 disease	
Cisplatin eligible	• Gemcitabine (Gemzar®, Infugem™) and cisplatin followed by avelumab (Bavencio®) maintenance therapy • Dose-dense methotrexate, vinblastine, doxorubicin, cisplatin (DDMVAC) with growth factor support and avelumab (Bavencio®) maintenance therapy
Cisplatin ineligible	• Gemcitabine (Gemzar®, Infugem™) and carboplatin followed by avelumab (Bavencio®) maintenance therapy (preferred) • Atezolizumab (Tecentriq®) (preferred) • Pembrolizumab (Keytruda®) (preferred) • Gemcitabine (Gemzar®, Infugem™) • Gemcitabine (Gemzar®, Infugem™) and paclitaxel (Taxol®) • Ifosfamide (Ifex®), doxorubicin, and gemcitabine (Gemzar®, Infugem™) (useful in certain circumstances)

Partial response

If you had a partial response to the systemic therapy, more treatment is needed.

Treatment may include:

> Surgery (radical cystectomy)

> Chemoradiotherapy

> Begin treatment for metastatic disease

Disease progression

Disease progression refers to no response to treatment. This means the cancer grew or spread. At this point you will begin treatment for metastatic disease.

Chemoradiation

Chemotherapy and radiation therapy are used together to try to kill the cancer. When given together, both treatments work better than either does alone. This option allows you to keep your bladder.

Within 2 to 3 months after treatment with systemic therapy, you will be tested to determine if the cancer responded to treatment. Tests may include CT imaging of the chest, abdomen, and/or pelvis with contrast.

Complete response

If you have a complete response to chemoradiation, no more treatment is needed. You can begin follow-up care and monitoring for cancer recurrence (return).

Partial response

If you have a partial response to chemoradiation, more treatment is needed.

Next treatment options include:

> Intravesical BCG therapy (if treatment succeeded at shrinking the tumor enough so that it no longer invades the muscle wall of the bladder)

> Surgery to remove what's left of the tumor

> Begin treatment for metastatic disease

No response

If your cancer did not respond to chemoradiation and the cancer grew or spread, you will begin treatment for metastatic disease.

Stage 4A

Some stage 4A bladder cancers have spread to distant lymph nodes or invade pelvic/abdominal walls. If the cancer has spread to distant lymph nodes, it is referred to as "M0" disease. If it spreads to distant lymph nodes, it is referred to as "M1a" disease.

Further testing is needed to identify which type of stage 4A cancer you have.

Tests may include:

> Abdominal or pelvic CT or MRI

> Chest imaging

> Bone scan

> Molecular or genomic testing

> Glomerular filtration rate (GRF) – to help determine eligibility for treatment with cisplatin

Treatment of all stage 4A bladder cancers starts out the same, but then differs based on whether there is cancer in distant lymph nodes. Treatment options are described next.

Non-metastatic disease
If testing shows that you have non-metastatic (M0) disease, you will be treated with one of the two following options:

> Systemic therapy

> Chemoradiotherapy

For a list of systemic therapy options, see Guide 4.

After treatment with systemic therapy or chemoradiotherapy, testing is needed to see if the cancer responded to treatment. Testing is recommended after 2 to 3 cycles of systemic therapy, or 2 to 3 months after finishing chemotherapy and radiation.

Tests will include:

> Cystoscopy

> Examination under anesthesia (EUA)

> TURBT

> Imaging tests of your abdomen and pelvis

If you had a complete response to treatment (no tumor is found) with either systemic therapy or chemoradiation, treatment options include:

> Systemic therapy

> Chemoradiotherapy (if you have not had RT)

> Cystectomy

Systemic therapy is used to kill any cancer cells that may still be in the body. This is referred to as consolidation systemic therapy. See Guide 4.

Chemoradiotherapy is a combination of radiation therapy (RT) and chemotherapy. This option is for people who have not had any radiation therapy previously. If you were treated with a low dose of RT, you may receive more.

Guide 5
Systemic therapy options: Stage 4

Post-platinum	• Pembrolizumab (Keytruda®) (preferred) • Paclitaxel (Taxol®) or docetaxel (Taxotere®) • Gemcitabine (Gemzar®, Infugem™) • Immune checkpoint inhibitors (Nivolumab [Opdivo®] or Avelumab [Bavencio®]) • Erdafitinib (Balversa®) • Ifosfamide (Ifex®), doxorubicin, and gemcitabine (Gemzar®, Infugem™) • Gemcitabine (Gemzar®, Infugem™) and cisplatin • DDMVAC with growth factor support
Post-checkpoint inhibitor	• Gemcitabine (Gemzar®, Infugem™) and carboplatin (preferred) • Erdafitinib (Balversa®) • Paclitaxel (Taxol®) or docetaxel (Taxotere®) • Gemcitabine (Gemzar®, Infugem™) • Gemcitabine (Gemzar®, Infugem™) and cisplatin • DDMVAC with growth factor support • Ifosfamide (Ifex®), doxorubicin, and gemcitabine (Gemzar®, Infugem™) • Gemcitabine (Gemzar®, Infugem™) and paclitaxel (Taxol®)
Post-platinum and maintenance therapy	• Enfortumab vedotin-ejfv (Padcev®) (preferred) • Erdafitinib (Balversa®) (preferred) • Gemcitabine (Gemzar®, Infugem™) • Paclitaxel (Taxol®) or docetaxel (Taxotere®) • Ifosfamide (Ifex®), doxorubicin, and gemcitabine (Gemzar®, Infugem™) • Gemcitabine (Gemzar®, Infugem™) and paclitaxel (Taxol®) • Gemcitabine (Gemzar®, Infugem™) and cisplatin • DDMVAC with growth factor support • Sacituzumab govitecan-hziy (Trodelvy®)

If testing shows that the tumor is still there, you may receive any of the following:

> Systemic therapy (see Guide 5)

> Chemoradiotherapy

> Cystectomy (surgery)

Metastatic disease

If you have metastatic (M1A) disease, you will be treated with systemic therapy. For a list of systemic therapy options, see Guide 5.

After being treated, you will be tested to determine if the tumor is gone.

You may receive the following tests:

> Cystoscopy

> Examination under anesthesia (EUA)

> TURBT

> Imaging of the abdomen and/or pelvis

If you have had a complete response (CR) to treatment and the tumor is gone, your doctor may ask you to consider local therapy (in certain cases). If your disease is stable or continues to spread, you will be treated as if you have metastatic disease.

Follow-up care

When you have finished treatment, the next phase of cancer care begins. This is the surveillance phase. During this time, it is important to have testing to monitor for the return of cancer. The specific tests you should have—and how often you should have them—depends on whether your bladder was removed.

Your bladder was removed

Follow-up after a radical cystectomy should include imaging studies, urine and blood tests, and liver and kidney function testing.

After the first year of follow-up care, your vitamin B12 level should be tested once per year. Urethral wash cytology is recommended during the first two years of follow-up care for those with high-risk disease who have an ileal conduit or a continent urinary reservoir.

Follow-up after a partial cystectomy is similar to that for a radical cystectomy. One difference is that after partial cystectomy, cytology and cystoscopy are recommended to look for signs that cancer has returned to the bladder.

You have your bladder

For those who were able to keep their bladder, there is a risk that cancer will recur (return). Follow-up tests look to see if the cancer has moved anywhere outside of the bladder in the urinary tract, or to areas far from the bladder.

Follow-up after bladder-preserving treatment should include cystoscopy, imaging studies, urine and blood tests, and liver and kidney function testing.

Recurrence or persistence

Cancer treatment for recurrence is based on results of tests as well as if your bladder was removed.

Specific tests include:

> Cytology

> Imaging

> Cystoscopy

You have your bladder
The following options are for those who have part or all of their bladder.

Muscle invasive tumors are usually treated in one of four ways:

> **Radical cystectomy.** This may not be possible if you have undergone a full course of EBRT and have a large tumor. In this case, best supportive care and TURBT to help relieve symptoms caused by the tumor are recommended.

> **Chemoradiotherapy.** This is an option for people who have not had any prior radiation therapy.

> **Palliative TURBT.** This is an option for people who have undergone a full course of EBRT and are not candidates for surgery. TURBT can be done to help relieve symptoms caused by the tumor. This is considered a palliative TURBT, because the goal is to make you more comfortable, not to cure the cancer.

> **Supportive care.** Supportive care is health care that relieves symptoms caused by cancer or its treatment and improves quality of life. It might include pain relief (palliative care), emotional or spiritual support, financial aid, or family counseling. Supportive care is given during all cancer stages. Speak to your care team about how you are feeling and any side effects.

Cancer has not responded to treatment (persistent disease)
In people with a preserved bladder, the treatment options for cancer that has not responded to treatment are the same as for cancer that returned to the bladder (or nearby). Treatment options depend on the size of the tumor and are explained next.

Cancer returned to the bladder (or nearby)
If cancer returns to the bladder (or nearby), it is called a local recurrence. It should be treated as a new cancer. Local recurrence tumors are treated based on the size of the tumor and treatments you have already received.

Non-muscle invasive tumors are usually treated with BCG therapy or radical cystectomy. If BCG therapy is used and doesn't work, radical cystectomy is recommended.

If you are not a candidate for surgery, options include:

> Chemoradiation (only if you haven't had any prior radiation therapy).

> Switching from BCG to a different intravesical medicine

> Joining a clinical trial

Follow-up urine cytology found cancer

If your test for cytology is positive, you will be asked to repeat the test within 3 months.

If your repeated cytology tests come back positive, you may be treated with the following:

> Intravesical bacillus Calmette-Guérin (BCG) therapy

> Cystectomy

> Pembrolizumab

Your bladder was removed

If your bladder was removed and cancer returned to the bladder area or metastasized (spread to distant areas), treatment options include:

> Systemic therapy

> Chemoradiotherapy (only if you have not had any radiation therapy to the area)

Radiation alone

This option may be helpful if the cancer has not spread far from the bladder or if the tumor is causing symptoms.

Key points

> If a bladder tumor grows large enough to reach the thick layer of muscle in the bladder wall, it is called muscle invasive bladder cancer. Stage 2, 3, and 4 bladder cancers are muscle invasive.

> In people healthy enough for surgery, the treatment options for stage 2 and 3A bladder cancer are cisplatin-based chemotherapy followed by radical cystectomy, and chemoradiation.

> The primary (main) treatment options for stage 3B and 4A bladder cancer are systemic therapy and chemoradiation.

> Follow-up testing after treatment for muscle invasive disease includes imaging tests, blood tests, and urine tests.

7
Metastatic (stage 4B)

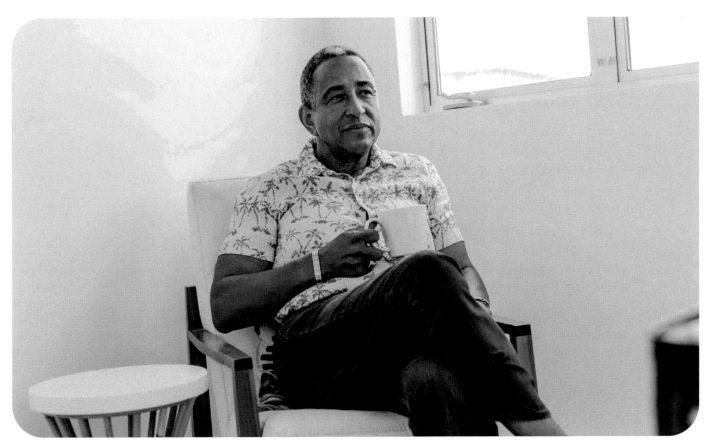

If cancer spreads to areas far from the bladder, it is called metastatic cancer. If it has already metastasized by the time you are diagnosed, it is stage 4B bladder cancer. Treatment of metastatic bladder cancer is focused on helping you live as normally and as comfortably as possible, for as long as possible.

Testing

If your cancer has spread beyond the pelvic region, you will receive further testing.

Tests may include:

> Bone scan (if your doctor thinks there may be cancer in your bones based on your symptoms or results of laboratory tests)

> CT of your chest

> Central nervous system (CNS) imaging

> Glomerular filtration rate (GRF) – to help determine eligibility for treatment with cisplatin

> Biopsy of any suspicious areas

> Molecular or genomic testing (to determine if there is a family history)

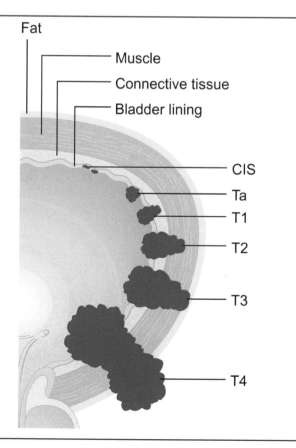

Stage 4 bladder cancer

In stage 4 bladder cancer, the tumor has grown through the bladder wall into surrounding areas.

Palliative RT

Palliative radiation therapy (RT) is used to ease pain or discomfort from bladder cancer. The RT does not aim to cure the cancer, so lower doses are used to reduce the occurrence of side effects. The goal of palliative RT is to control cancer symptoms or stop them in order to provide a better quality of life.

Systemic therapy

The main treatment for metastatic bladder cancer is systemic therapy. Systemic therapy includes chemotherapy, targeted therapy, and immunotherapy medicines. In order to determine which systemic therapy medicines are best for you, your doctor will consider your overall health. This includes how your heart, liver, and kidneys are functioning, how far the cancer has progressed, and your ability to do day-to-day activities.

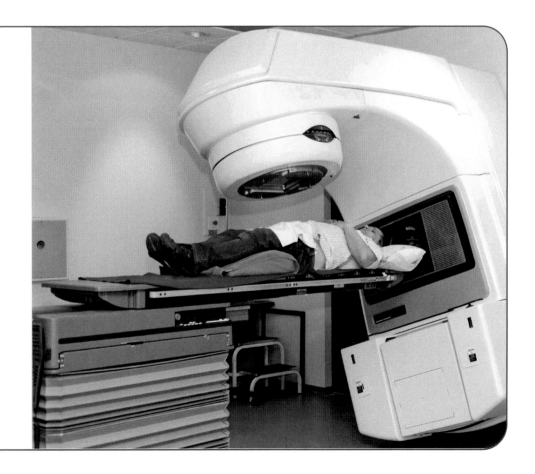

Radiation therapy

A man is shown receiving radiation therapy.

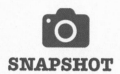

SNAPSHOT

Systemic therapy for metastatic bladder cancer

Platinum-based chemotherapy

cisplatin

carboplatin

- The standard of care for metastatic bladder cancer

- Given in combination with other chemotherapy agents

- Cisplatin and carboplatin are platinum-based chemotherapies

- Cisplatin is the stronger drug in terms of response and side effects

- This type of chemotherapy (especially cisplatin) can damage the kidneys

- Many people can't have cisplatin because their kidneys don't work well or because of other health issues

Checkpoint inhibitors

pembrolizumab (Keytruda®)

atezolizumab (Tecentriq®)

nivolumab (Opdivo®)

enfortumab vedotin-ejfv (Padcev®)

avelumab (Bavencio®)

- Checkpoint inhibitors are a newer treatment option for locally advanced and metastatic bladder cancer

- Some can be used for bladder cancer that progresses or metastasizes after platinum-based chemotherapy

- Some can also be used as first-line therapy for people with the PD-L1 biomarker who can't have cisplatin, and for people who can't have any platinum-based chemotherapy

FGFR inhibitor

erdafitinib (Balversa™)

- New treatment option for some people with *FGFR2* or *FGFR3* mutations

- For people with locally advanced or metastatic disease who have progressed on platinum-based chemotherapy

- Given as a once-daily pill

Other systemic therapies

- There are other systemic therapy regimens that may be helpful.

- NCCN experts recommend joining a clinical trial if there is one available to you.

Supportive care

Supportive care is health care that relieves symptoms caused by cancer or its treatment and improves quality of life. It might include pain relief (palliative care), emotional or spiritual support, financial aid, or family counseling. Supportive care is given during all cancer stages. Tell your care team how you are feeling and about any side effects. Best supportive care is used with other treatments to improve quality of life. Best supportive care, supportive care, and palliative care are often used interchangeably.

Distress

Distress is an unpleasant experience of a mental, physical, social, or spiritual nature. It can affect how you feel, think, and act. Distress might include feelings of sadness, fear, helplessness, worry, anger, and guilt. You may also experience depression, anxiety, and sleeping problems.

For more information, read *NCCN Guidelines for Patients: Distress During Cancer Care*, available at NCCN.org/patientguidelines.

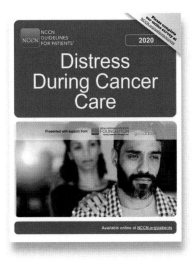

Side effects

Treatment of bladder cancer can cause unwanted changes to your body and mind, called side effects. Some side effects can be harmful to your health, while others are just unpleasant. The effects of treatment depend on many factors, especially the treatment type (radiation versus chemotherapy, for example) and the length or dose of the treatment. Side effects can last for years; some may never go away.

Side effects may include:

> **Sexual dysfunction.** This includes a decreased desire to have sex. This may be due to a lack of energy, being self-conscious about your body after surgery, or feeling stressed out and depressed.

> **Trouble controlling the flow of urine.** This is referred to as urinary incontinence. Urine may come out when you do not want it or expect it to, including during sex.

Sexual dysfunction and urinary incontinence are only two examples of side effects. Ask your treatment team for a complete list of short- and long-term side effects and information on how to manage them. Many side effects can be managed. Some may even be preventable.

Key points

> You should expect further testing if the cancer has spread beyond the bladder walls.

> The main treatment for metastatic bladder cancer is systemic therapy.

> Systemic therapy includes chemotherapy, targeted therapy, and immunotherapy.

> Palliative radiation therapy (RT) is used to ease pain or discomfort from bladder cancer.

> Supportive care aims to improve your quality of life. It includes care for health issues caused by cancer or cancer treatment.

You may receive blood and urine tests to show how well the kidneys are working. Kidneys help to remove waste from the body.

8
Making treatment decisions

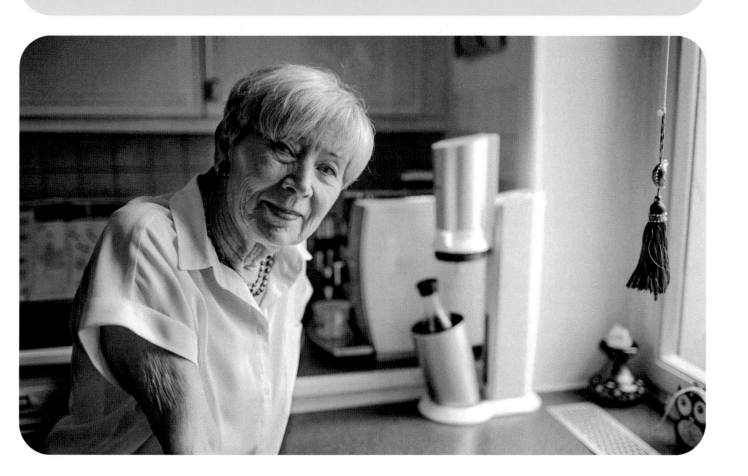

It's important to be comfortable with the cancer treatment you choose. This choice starts with having an open and honest conversation with your doctor.

It's your choice

In shared decision-making, you and your doctors share information, discuss the options, and agree on a treatment plan. It starts with an open and honest conversation between you and your doctor.

Treatment decisions are very personal. What is important to you may not be important to someone else.

Some things that may play a role in your decision-making:

> What you want and how that might differ from what others want

> Your religious and spiritual beliefs

> Your feelings about certain treatments like surgery or chemotherapy

> Your feelings about pain or side effects such as nausea and vomiting

> Cost of treatment, travel to treatment centers, and time away from work

> Quality of life and length of life

> How active you are and the activities that are important to you

Think about what you want from treatment. Discuss openly the risks and benefits of specific treatments and procedures. Weigh options and share concerns with your doctor. If you take the time to build a relationship with your doctor, it will help you feel supported when considering options and making treatment decisions.

Second opinion

It is normal to want to start treatment as soon as possible. While cancer can't be ignored, there is time to have another doctor review your test results and suggest a treatment plan. This is called getting a second opinion, and it's a normal part of cancer care. Even doctors get second opinions!

Things you can do to prepare:

> Check with your insurance company about its rules on second opinions. There may be out-of-pocket costs to see doctors who are not part of your insurance plan.

> Make plans to have copies of all your records sent to the doctor you will see for your second opinion.

Support groups

Many people diagnosed with cancer find support groups to be helpful. Support groups often include people at different stages of treatment. Some people may be newly diagnosed, while others may be finished with treatment. If your hospital or community doesn't have support groups for people with cancer, check out the websites listed in this book.

Questions to ask your doctors

Possible questions to ask your doctors are listed on the following pages. Feel free to use these or come up with your own. Be clear about your goals for treatment and find out what to expect from treatment.

Questions to ask about diagnosis and testing

1. What type of bladder cancer do I have?

2. What tests do I need?

3. Who will perform these tests? Where will they be done?

4. Are there any complications from these tests?

5. Do the tests hurt?

6. When will I get the test results? How will you inform me?

7. What is the chance of recurrence?

8. Is it possible to develop cancer elsewhere in my body?

9. What stage and grade is my cancer? What does this mean?

10. Does my insurance cover testing and treatment? Who can help me find out more about this?

Questions to ask about options

1. Will my age, health, and other factors affect my options?

2. Am I a candidate for a clinical trial?

3. Do you participate in clinical trials?

4. May I have a copy of my test results?

5. What should I do on weekends and other non-office hours if I get a fever, have another reaction, or have a side effect from cancer or cancer treatment? Where should I go?

6. What support services are available to me?

7. Are there any other therapies I can do while receiving cancer treatment?

Questions to ask about treatment

1. What are my treatment options?

2. How soon will I be treated?

3. Where will I be treated?

4. What is the goal of each treatment?

5. What are the treatment side effects? Long-term and short-term?

6. Are there any complications from treatment?

7. What are the chances that my cancer can be cured?

8. If my bladder is removed, what are my options for passing urine?

9. Will treatment for my cancer affect my fertility? What are my options to protect it?

10. How long will treatment last?

11. Will treatment affect my daily activities?

12. What do we do if the cancer returns?

Questions to ask about the surgery

1. Why do I need surgery?

2. What procedure will I receive?

3. How soon will the surgery take place?

4. What are the risks and benefits of this surgery?

5. Are there any nonsurgical options?

6. Are there less invasive surgery options?

7. What happens if the surgery does not work for me?

Questions to ask your doctors about their experience

1. Who will be part of my health care team, and what does each member do?

2. Who will be leading my overall treatment?

3. What is your experience in treating people with bladder cancer?

4. Who else will be on my treatment team?

5. Do I need to see any other health care providers?

6. Are you board certified?

Websites

American Bladder Cancer Society
bladdercancersupport.org

American Cancer Society®
cancer.org/cancer/bladder-cancer.html

American Lung Association
lung.org/quit-smoking/join-freedom-from-smoking

Bladder Cancer Advocacy Network
bcan.org

National Cancer Institute
cancer.gov/types/bladder

National Coalition for Cancer Survivorship
canceradvocacy.org/toolbox

National Hospice and Palliative Care Organization
nhpco.org/patients-and-caregivers

Urology Care Foundation
urologyhealth.org

U.S. Centers for Disease Control & Prevention
cdc.gov/tobacco/quit_smoking/index.htm

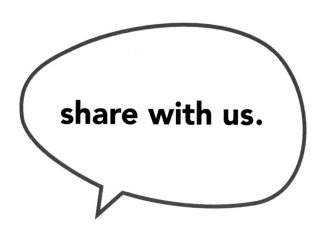

Take our survey and help make the NCCN Guidelines for Patients better for everyone!

NCCN.org/patients/comments

Words to know

bacillus Calmette Guérin (BCG)
An immunotherapy medicine put directly into the bladder to treat bladder cancer.

benign tumor
A tumor that can grow but will not spread.

biomarker
Any molecule in your body that can be measured to assess your health. Usually identified by a test done on your tumor tissue or a blood test.

biopsy
A procedure that removes fluid or tissue samples to be tested for disease.

bone scan
A test that makes pictures of bones to assess for health problems.

cancer grade
A rating of how much the cancer cells look like normal cells under a microscope and how aggressive the cancer is.

cancer stage
A rating of the outlook of a cancer based on its growth and spread.

carcinoma in situ (CIS)
Flat, high-grade (fast-growing) tumors.

chemoradiation
Cancer treatment with both chemotherapy and radiation therapy.

chemotherapy
Cancer drugs that stop the cell life cycle to kill the cancer cells.

clinical stage
The rating of the extent of cancer before surgery.

clinical trials
A type of research that assesses how well health tests or treatments work in people.

complete blood count (CBC)
A common blood test that provides information about the numbers and kinds of cells in the blood, especially red blood cells, white blood cells, and platelets.

computed tomography (CT)
A test that uses x-rays from many angles to make a picture of the insides of the body.

computed tomography urogram (CTU)
An imaging method that uses x-rays to create detailed pictures of the kidneys, ureters, and bladder.

consolidation therapy
A treatment given after the cancer is gone in order to kill any last cancer cells that may be hiding in the body. Also called intensification therapy and post-remission therapy.

continent urinary reservoir
A type of urinary diversion in which a piece of intestine is used to make a small reservoir in the wall of the abdomen. A catheter is used to drain urine from the reservoir. Also called an Indiana pouch and a continent catheterizable diversion.

cystectomy
A surgical procedure that removes all or part of the bladder.

cystoscopy
A procedure that allows a doctor to see inside the bladder using a special tool inserted through the urethra. Usually occurs in the doctor's regular office in a procedure room.

dose-dense chemotherapy
A method of speeding up chemotherapy by reducing the amount of time between treatments.

dose-dense methotrexate, vinblastine, doxorubicin, and cisplatin (DDMVAC)
A chemotherapy regimen used to treat bladder cancer.

examination under anesthesia (EUA)
An examination of a specific area of the body while the patient is under general anesthesia.

external beam radiation therapy (EBRT)
A cancer treatment with radiation delivered from a machine outside the body.

glomerular filtration rate (GFR)
The flow rate of filtered fluid through the kidneys to assess the function of the kidneys before giving cisplatin-based chemotherapy.

growth factor
A substance that helps new blood cells to be made. Used to help the blood cells recover between rounds of chemotherapy.

hematuria
The presence of blood in urine.

hydronephrosis
Abnormal enlargement (swelling) of a kidney caused by a build-up of urine. In cancer, this can be caused by an obstruction from the tumor growth.

ileal conduit
A type of urinary diversion in which a piece of small intestine is used as a pipeline (conduit) for urine to leave the body through a hole (stoma) in the abdomen.

immunotherapy
Treatment with drugs that help the body's immune system find and destroy cancer cells.

instillation
A method used to slowly put liquid into the body.

intravesical therapy
A treatment using medicine put directly into the bladder.

lamina propria
A layer of connective tissue within the wall of the urinary tract.

locally advanced cancer
Cancer that has spread from the first site to nearby tissue or lymph nodes.

local therapy
A treatment that is given to a specific area or organ of the body.

magnetic resonance imaging (MRI)
An imaging method that uses radio waves and powerful magnets to make pictures of the insides of the body.

magnetic resonance urogram (MRU)
An imaging method that uses magnetic waves to create detailed pictures of the kidneys, ureters, and bladder.

malignant
A tumor that can grow and spread to other parts of the body.

medical history
A report of all your health events and medications.

muscularis propria
The third layer of the wall of the urinary tract. Also called the detrusor muscle.

mutation
An abnormal change in the coded instructions within cells.

neobladder
A type of urinary diversion in which a piece of small intestine is made into a hollow pouch that can hold and drain urine.

observation
A period of testing for changes in cancer status while not receiving treatment.

pathologic stage
A rating of the extent of cancer based on tests given after surgery to treat the primary tumor.

positron emission tomography (PET)
A test that uses radioactive material to see the shape and function of body parts.

primary treatment
The main treatment used to rid the body of cancer.

radiation therapy
A treatment that uses intense energy to kill cancer cells.

radical cystectomy
A surgical procedure that removes the bladder, nearby lymph nodes, and other organs in the pelvis.

radiosensitization
The use of a drug that makes tumor cells more sensitive to radiation therapy.

radiosensitizing agent
Any substance that makes tumor cells easier to kill with radiation therapy. Some radiosensitizing agents are being studied in the treatment of cancer. Also called radiosensitizer.

recurrence
The return of cancer after a cancer-free period.

supportive care
Health care that includes symptom relief but not cancer treatment. Also called palliative care.

surveillance
Testing that is done after treatment ends to look for new tumors.

systemic therapy
A type of treatment that works throughout the body.

targeted therapy
A cancer treatment that may target and attack specific types of cancer cells.

transurethral resection of the bladder tumor (TURBT)
A procedure to remove bladder tumors via the urethra. Determines the tumor stage of bladder cancer.

ureter
A long, tube-shaped structure that carries urine from the kidneys to the bladder.

ureteroscopy
A procedure that allows a doctor to see inside the kidney and ureter using a special tool called a uteroscope. The uteroscope is inserted into the urethra and then guided through the bladder, ureter, and into the kidney.

urinary diversion
A type of surgery that creates a new way for urine to leave the body after radical cystectomy.

urine cytology
A lab test performed on urine to detect disease.

urothelium
The stretchy lining of the organs of the urinary tract. This includes the kidneys, ureters, bladder, and urethra.

NCCN Contributors

This patient guide is based on the NCCN Clinical Practice Guidelines in Oncology (NCCN Guidelines®) for Bladder Cancer, Version 3.2021 — April 22, 2021. It was adapted, reviewed, and published with help from the following people:

Dorothy A. Shead, MS
Senior Director
Patient Information Operations

Rachael Clarke
Senior Medical Copyeditor

Tanya Fischer, MEd, MSLIS
Medical Writer

Laura J. Hanisch, PsyD
Program Manager
Patient Information Operations

Stephanie Helbling, MPH, MCHES®
Medical Writer

Susan Kidney
Senior Graphic Design Specialist

John Murphy
Medical Writer

Jeanette Shultz
Patient Guidelines Coordinator

Erin Vidic, MA
Medical Writer

Kim Williams
Creative Services Manager

NCCN Clinical Practice Guidelines in Oncology (NCCN Guidelines®) for Bladder Cancer, Version 3.2021 — April 22, 2021 were developed by the following NCCN Panel Members:

Thomas W. Flaig, MD
University of Colorado Cancer Center

Philippe E. Spiess, MD, MS
Moffitt Cancer Center

*Neeraj Agarwal, MD
Huntsman Cancer Institute
at the University of Utah

*Rick Bangs, MBA
Patient Advocate

Stephen A. Boorjian, MD
Mayo Clinic Cancer Center

Mark K. Buyyounouski, MD, MS
Stanford Cancer Institute

*Kevin Chan, MD
City of Hope National Medical Center

Sam Chang, MD, MBA
Vanderbilt-Ingram Cancer Center

Tracy M. Downs, MD
University of Wisconsin
Carbone Cancer Center

Terence Friedlander, MD
UCSF Helen Diller Family
Comprehensive Cancer Center

Richard E. Greenberg, MD
Fox Chase Cancer Center

Khurshid A. Guru, MD
Roswell Park Comprehensive Cancer Center

Thomas Guzzo, MD, MPH
Abramson Cancer Center
at the University of Pennsylvania

Harry W. Herr, MD
Memorial Sloan Kettering Cancer Center

Jean Hoffman-Censits, MD
The Sidney Kimmel Comprehensive
Cancer Center at Johns Hopkins

Brant A. Inman, MD, MSc
Duke Cancer Institute

Masahito Jimbo, MD, PhD, MPH
University of Michigan Rogel Cancer Center

A. Karim Kader, MD, PhD
UC San Diego Moores Cancer Center

Amar Kishan, MD
UCLA Jonsson
Comprehensive Cancer Center

Subodh M. Lele, MD
Fred & Pamela Buffett Cancer Center

Vitaly Margulis, MD
UT Southwestern Simmons Comprehensive
Cancer Center

Omar Y. Mian, MD, PhD
Case Comprehensive Cancer Center/
University Hospitals Seidman Cancer
Center and Cleveland Clinic Taussig
Cancer Institute

Jeff Michalski, MD, MBA
Siteman Cancer Center at Barnes-
Jewish Hospital and Washington
University School of Medicine

Jeffrey S. Montgomery, MD, MHSA
University of Michigan Rogel Cancer Center

Lakshminarayanan Nandagopal, MD
O'Neal Comprehensive
Cancer Center at UAB

Lance C. Pagliaro, MD
Mayo Clinic Cancer Center

*Anthony Patterson, MD
St. Jude Children's Research Hospital/
The University of Tennessee
Health Science Center

Elizabeth R. Plimack, MD, MS
Fox Chase Cancer Center

Kamal S. Pohar, MD
The Ohio State University Comprehensive
Cancer Center - James Cancer Hospital
and Solove Research Institute

Mark A. Preston, MD, MPH
Dana-Farber/Brigham and Women's
Cancer Center

Wade J. Sexton, MD
Moffitt Cancer Center

Arlene O. Siefker-Radtke, MD
The University of Texas
MD Anderson Cancer Center

Jonathan Tward, MD, PhD
Huntsman Cancer Institute
at the University of Utah

Jonathan L. Wright, MD, MS
Fred Hutchinson Cancer Research Center/
Seattle Cancer Care Alliance

NCCN Staff

Lisa Gurski, PhD

Mary Dwyer, MS

* Reviewed this patient guide.
For disclosures, visit NCCN.org/disclosures.

NCCN Cancer Centers

Abramson Cancer Center
at the University of Pennsylvania
Philadelphia, Pennsylvania
800.789.7366 • pennmedicine.org/cancer

Fred & Pamela Buffett Cancer Center
Omaha, Nebraska
402.559.5600 • unmc.edu/cancercenter

Case Comprehensive Cancer Center/
University Hospitals Seidman Cancer
Center and Cleveland Clinic Taussig
Cancer Institute
Cleveland, Ohio
800.641.2422 • UH Seidman Cancer Center
uhhospitals.org/services/cancer-services
866.223.8100 • CC Taussig Cancer Institute
my.clevelandclinic.org/departments/cancer
216.844.8797 • Case CCC
case.edu/cancer

City of Hope National Medical Center
Los Angeles, California
800.826.4673 • cityofhope.org

Dana-Farber/Brigham and
Women's Cancer Center |
Massachusetts General Hospital
Cancer Center
Boston, Massachusetts
617.732.5500
youhaveus.org
617.726.5130
massgeneral.org/cancer-center

Duke Cancer Institute
Durham, North Carolina
888.275.3853 • dukecancerinstitute.org

Fox Chase Cancer Center
Philadelphia, Pennsylvania
888.369.2427 • foxchase.org

Huntsman Cancer Institute
at the University of Utah
Salt Lake City, Utah
800.824.2073
huntsmancancer.org

Fred Hutchinson Cancer
Research Center/Seattle
Cancer Care Alliance
Seattle, Washington
206.606.7222 • seattlecca.org
206.667.5000 • fredhutch.org

The Sidney Kimmel Comprehensive
Cancer Center at Johns Hopkins
Baltimore, Maryland
410.955.8964
www.hopkinskimmelcancercenter.org

Robert H. Lurie Comprehensive
Cancer Center of Northwestern
University
Chicago, Illinois
866.587.4322 • cancer.northwestern.edu

Mayo Clinic Cancer Center
Phoenix/Scottsdale, Arizona
Jacksonville, Florida
Rochester, Minnesota
480.301.8000 • Arizona
904.953.0853 • Florida
507.538.3270 • Minnesota
mayoclinic.org/cancercenter

Memorial Sloan Kettering
Cancer Center
New York, New York
800.525.2225 • mskcc.org

Moffitt Cancer Center
Tampa, Florida
888.663.3488 • moffitt.org

The Ohio State University
Comprehensive Cancer Center -
James Cancer Hospital and
Solove Research Institute
Columbus, Ohio
800.293.5066 • cancer.osu.edu

O'Neal Comprehensive
Cancer Center at UAB
Birmingham, Alabama
800.822.0933 • uab.edu/onealcancercenter

Roswell Park Comprehensive
Cancer Center
Buffalo, New York
877.275.7724 • roswellpark.org

Siteman Cancer Center at Barnes-
Jewish Hospital and Washington
University School of Medicine
St. Louis, Missouri
800.600.3606 • siteman.wustl.edu

St. Jude Children's Research Hospital/
The University of Tennessee
Health Science Center
Memphis, Tennessee
866.278.5833 • stjude.org
901.448.5500 • uthsc.edu

Stanford Cancer Institute
Stanford, California
877.668.7535 • cancer.stanford.edu

UC Davis
Comprehensive Cancer Center
Sacramento, California
916.734.5959 • 800.770.9261
health.ucdavis.edu/cancer

UC San Diego Moores Cancer Center
La Jolla, California
858.822.6100 • cancer.ucsd.edu

UCLA Jonsson
Comprehensive Cancer Center
Los Angeles, California
310.825.5268 • cancer.ucla.edu

UCSF Helen Diller Family
Comprehensive Cancer Center
San Francisco, California
800.689.8273 • cancer.ucsf.edu

University of Colorado Cancer Center
Aurora, Colorado
720.848.0300 • coloradocancercenter.org

University of Michigan
Rogel Cancer Center
Ann Arbor, Michigan
800.865.1125 • rogelcancercenter.org

The University of Texas
MD Anderson Cancer Center
Houston, Texas
844.269.5922 • mdanderson.org

University of Wisconsin
Carbone Cancer Center
Madison, Wisconsin
608.265.1700 • uwhealth.org/cancer

UT Southwestern Simmons
Comprehensive Cancer Center
Dallas, Texas
214.648.3111 • utsouthwestern.edu/simmons

Vanderbilt-Ingram Cancer Center
Nashville, Tennessee
877.936.8422 • vicc.org

Yale Cancer Center/
Smilow Cancer Hospital
New Haven, Connecticut
855.4.SMILOW • yalecancercenter.org

Notes

Index

Manufactured by Amazon.ca
Bolton, ON

25637147R00048